BUSTING THE CODE TO AGEING:
HOW TO WIN THE INFLAMMATION GAME

Dr Victoria Manning

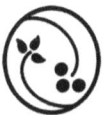

First published 2025
by Rowanvale Books Ltd
The Gate
Keppoch Street
Roath
Cardiff
CF24 3JW
www.rowanvalebooks.com

A CIP catalogue record for this book is available from the British Library.
ISBN: 978-1-83584-090-0
eBook ISBN: 978-1-83584-091-7

To Paul Trevorrow, my husband, who has stood beside me through every research rabbit-hole, late-night writing session and 'just one more chapter' moment. Your patience with my passion for understanding ageing and inflammation knows no bounds. Thank you for being my constant support and occasional test subject.

To my incredible team at River Aesthetics, your enthusiasm, professionalism and willingness to grow have made every day an adventure. Thank you for believing in this vision and helping bring it to life through your dedicated patient care.

Together, you have all made this book possible.

CONTENTS

THE HIDDEN FLAME

Epigraph by Dr Victoria Manning

Beneath the surface of our ageing skin,
A quiet fire burns, deep within,
Day by day, year after year,
Making our youth slowly disappear.
Like embers glowing in the night,
Inflammation dims our youthful light.
Breaking down what makes us new,
Collagen, elastin bid adieu.
In every wrinkle, every line,
We see these flames leave their design,
But understanding how they burn
Gives doctors power, helps us learn.
For in our quest to keep time still,
We must first know what makes us ill.
This wisdom guides our healing art,
As we give ageing a fresh start.
Whether doctor, patient, young or old,
These pages make hard science gold.
Simple truths for all to see,
The gift of knowledge, flowing free.

INTRODUCTION

Have you ever thought about how important it is to invest in your health? Well, now is the time! According to the World Health Organisation (WHO), the average person spends the last 20% of their life in poor health—that's about 16 years. As a medical professional and founder of DOSED by Doctors skincare, I've dedicated my career to changing this statistic, one person at a time.

What fascinates me most is how our understanding of ageing has evolved. In 2019, the World Health Organization added "ageing-related diseases" to its International Classification of Diseases, recognising ageing as a major risk factor for numerous health conditions. This breakthrough has transformed how we approach anti-ageing treatments, especially in dermatology and preventive medicine.

After two decades in medicine, first as a GP and now as an aesthetic doctor, I discovered something that's transforming how we think about ageing. While examining thousands of faces and treating countless skin conditions, a pattern emerged that has changed my entire approach to age management: inflammation isn't just a side effect of ageing, it's one of its primary drivers.

This discovery didn't happen overnight. It came from years of observing how some patients seem to age more rapidly than others, despite similar lifestyles, and from noticing how patients with certain health conditions experience accelerated ageing, while others maintain remarkable vitality well into their later years.

The common thread? Their inflammatory status.

What you're reading isn't just another anti-ageing book. It's the culmination of twenty years of clinical observation, cutting-edge research and breakthrough discoveries into how inflammation influences every aspect of how we age. Understanding this connection has revolutionised my practice, transformed my patients' results and could fundamentally change how you think about ageing.

Have I gained your attention?

It is not just the visible signs of ageing that we need to worry about – chronic inflammation can lead to a range of skin conditions including acne, rosacea, eczema and psoriasis. Whether you're dealing with a specific skin concern, interested in prevention or simply curious about the science behind inflammation, you'll find practical, actionable information in this book.

Your decision to embark on this journey alongside me marks the beginning of what I hope will be a fulfilling and fun exploration into the intricacies of your skin health and ageing. While there are countless skincare guides out there, I promise to make this journey different – I believe in making complex topics digestible and even enjoyable.

What makes inflammation so fascinating is its dual nature; it is both an internal timekeeper and a response to external assaults. Modern medicine often treats symptoms in isolation, but inflammation demands a comprehensive approach. My goal, as both a practising physician and skincare entrepreneur, is to empower you with science-backed strategies to transform your skin health. In the following chapters, we'll explore inflammation from every angle – medical, practical and personal. You'll learn how to identify different types of inflammation, understand their triggers and master practical strategies to maintain your skin's health. From dietary choices to skincare ingredients, stress management to exercise routines, we'll cover everything you need to know to take control of your skin's future.

Throughout this book, I have decoded complex science into actionable steps, bridging the gap between clinical research and practical, everyday solutions and helping you make informed decisions about your approach to skincare. These insights have revolutionised how I treat patients, and now I'm excited to share them with you.

On our journey, you'll find two special features I've included to make the science more accessible and personally relevant:

#PersonalTales – Because sometimes the best way to understand complex medical concepts is through real-life experiences. I'll share candid stories from my own journey and clinical practice, from my struggles with sleep (those Princess Leia headphones!) to what I've learned from treating thousands of patients.

#DrVixTakeaways – At the end of each chapter, you'll find five key points that summarise the complex information into practical, actionable insights. Think of these as your quick-reference guide to the most important concepts we've covered – perfect for when you need a rapid refresh.

Let's begin this journey of understanding how inflammation shapes our ageing process and, more importantly, what we can do about it.

This matters because, recall those 16 years of poor health we mentioned? They're not set in stone. By understanding and managing inflammation, you're not just investing in better-looking skin – you're investing in your overall health and longevity.

Think of this book as your friendly guide to understanding and managing skin ageing. Together, we'll uncover the secrets to maintaining healthy, vibrant skin at any age. And who knows? You might even enjoy learning the science behind it all!

ABOUT THE AUTHOR

If you'd told me in medical school that I'd end up writing a book about inflammation while running three aesthetic clinics and a skincare company, I'd have probably choked on my wine. My path to becoming an anti-inflammatory-skincare doctor wasn't conventional – but, then again, whose life story ever is?

My journey began at Southampton University in 1996, where I took a rather 'creative' approach to my education. Thanks to my late husband's airline connections, I found myself frequently escaping to Beirut for weekend ski trips and pool days, much to my pathology tutor's disbelief. So, getting to medical school itself was a battle – after a less-than-stellar physics grade landed me reading Physiology and Biochemistry, I practically haunted the medical dean's office until he offered me a challenge: achieve a first in my end-of-year exams to transfer to medicine. Challenge accepted.

Post-graduation, life took unexpected turns. A naval medical cadetship was cut short by a heart condition, leading me to general practice. Then came the defining moment – 5 October 1999 at St Mary's Hospital, when the Paddington train crash victims began arriving. That day taught me more about medicine and humanity than any textbook ever could.

Rural Shropshire followed, where I became a GP partner and women's health specialist. Small-town medicine brought its own adventures – trying to convince patients that the vegetable aisle wasn't ideal for discussing intimate health concerns became a regular occurrence.

But everything changed in 2009 when I lost my husband to suicide at thirty-seven, leaving me juggling two young children, a career in medicine and a household that often felt more like a circus act than a family. Overnight, my life shifted from 'married doctor' to 'single parent in a permanent state of organised chaos'. I became a one-woman show, complete with hastily packed lunches, bedtime negotiations and occasional tears (mostly mine).

This led me into addiction medicine, which taught me that healing doesn't come with a simple prescription pad. It's a mix of compassion, patience and, occasionally, the ability to keep a straight face when patients – true characters in their own right – explain the elaborate stories behind their latest 'mishaps'. This chapter brought me new perspectives, a bit of laughter in the face of adversity and a deep understanding that, sometimes, the best medicine is just showing up, rain or shine, with an open mind and a sense of humour firmly intact.

Then came my five-year stint as a prison doctor – armed with my own set of keys and my now robust sense of humour. The male prison environment brought unique challenges, particularly an inexplicable surge in genital-related consultations once word spread about the new female GP. Let's just say my medical expertise wasn't the only thing in high demand!

However, when the prison demographic shifted toward more serious offenders, I knew it was time for change.

In 2013, I took the biggest leap – co-founding an aesthetic clinic while being a single mother. Every penny mattered, and failure wasn't an option. Those early days were a blur of coffee-fuelled determination and 3 a.m. anxiety attacks, but the risk paid off. The clinic grew exponentially, gaining national recognition and, eventually, international acclaim. We found ourselves at the forefront of aesthetic innovation, particularly in the realms of thread-lifting techniques and collagen-stimulation protocols, eventually leading to successful acquisition by a private equity company in 2023.

My own health journey became intertwined with my professional evolution. A reality check came in the form of a conference photo – no clever angles or poses could hide what years of neglecting my own health looked like. Like many doctors, I'd mastered the art of helping others while completely overlooking my own wellbeing. This wake-up call, along with mounting aches and inflammation issues, pushed me to deep dive into metabolic health research. Sometimes, we doctors make the worst patients – but at least we know where to look for solutions!

My journey from size 16 to 12 taught me invaluable lessons about weight, inflammation and overall health, and it was this personal transformation that led me to explore inflammation from every angle. While my aesthetic clinic successfully treats the visible signs of ageing – addressing skin quality, volume loss and sagging – I became increasingly aware that true health optimisation requires a more comprehensive, holistic approach.

Most recently, I've ventured into test-based nutrition and developed my own skincare line, focusing on inflammation's role in ageing. With fewer than 700 dermatologists serving the UK's population of 70 million, there's a critical need for science-based information about skin health and inflammation.

This book emerges from that need – combining professional expertise with personal experience to understand inflammation's role in health and ageing. Think of it as your guide to understanding and managing inflammation, written by someone who's experienced it from every perspective – doctor, patient and skincare formulator.

The journey ahead might challenge some of your existing beliefs about health and ageing, but I promise it will be worth it.

PROLOGUE

The Fire Within: Understanding Inflammation and 'Inflammageing'

Understanding the Inflammation-Ageing Connection.

Think of inflammation as your body's internal alarm system – when something's not right, it sends out signals to protect you. In small doses, like a careful friend watching your back, inflammation helps defend your body, but when this alarm system stays on too long, that's when the trouble begins.

Over time, constant inflammation causes the skin to wear and tear, lose its elasticity and show signs of damage. This process – where chronic, low-grade inflammation accelerates how quickly our skin ages – is what we call 'inflammageing'. This isn't just another theory; it's a revolutionary understanding that's transforming how we approach longevity and health.

In youth, inflammation is your faithful guardian, swiftly responding to threats and healing injuries. When you cut your finger or catch a cold, acute inflammation swoops in – your blood vessels dilate, immune cells rush to the scene and healing begins. But as time passes, this protective response can become your biggest adversary, smouldering quietly beneath the surface, accelerating the very ageing process it once protected against – swift, purposeful but sometimes a bit overzealous.

Understanding this process is the foundation upon which all other aspects of ageing and wellness build. This is where our journey begins.

The Good Fight: Acute Inflammation.

Your acute inflammatory response is a masterpiece of biological engineering. Within seconds of injury or infection, your body launches a cascade of events that would make a military strategist proud.

The first responders, called neutrophils, arrive within minutes, followed by macrophages. You can think of them as the clean-up crew (or Pac-Man) that also calls for backup when needed. This process is choreographed by tiny molecular messengers called cytokines, your body's group chat, rapidly spreading the word about where help is needed.

Cytokines, like interleukin-6 (IL-6) and tumour necrosis factor-alpha (TNF-α), send out SOS signals that cause blood vessels to become more permeable, creating the familiar signs of acute inflammation: redness, swelling, heat and, sometimes, pain – all signs that your body is actively fighting and healing.

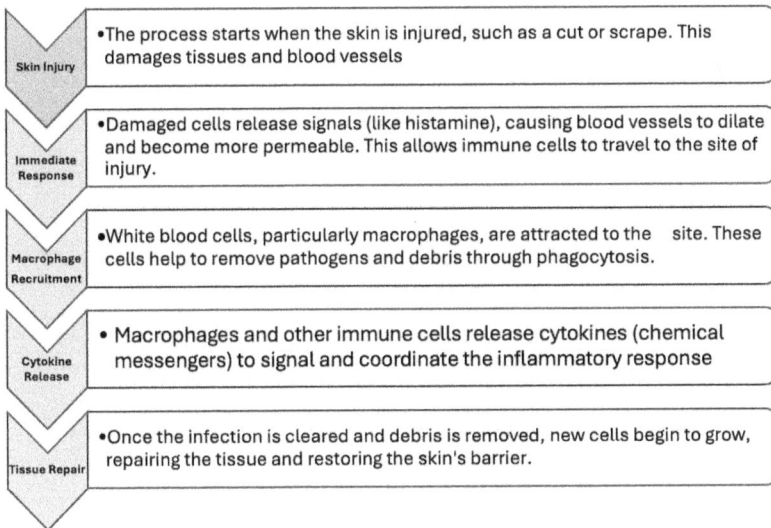

Skin Injury	•The process starts when the skin is injured, such as a cut or scrape. This damages tissues and blood vessels
Immediate Response	•Damaged cells release signals (like histamine), causing blood vessels to dilate and become more permeable. This allows immune cells to travel to the site of injury.
Macrophage Recruitment	•White blood cells, particularly macrophages, are attracted to the site. These cells help to remove pathogens and debris through phagocytosis.
Cytokine Release	• Macrophages and other immune cells release cytokines (chemical messengers) to signal and coordinate the inflammatory response
Tissue Repair	•Once the infection is cleared and debris is removed, new cells begin to grow, repairing the tissue and restoring the skin's barrier.

The Accute Inflammatory Response

When the Guards Won't Stand Down: Chronic Inflammation. But here's where it gets interesting: sometimes this emergency response team camps out indefinitely, causing collateral damage along the way. That's chronic inflammation. Your cytokines, once helpful messengers, become like that friend who won't stop sending notifications in the group chat. They keep recruiting immune cells, maintaining a constant state of alert that can silently damage your tissues.

This persistent state of inflammation creates a vicious cycle. Your immune cells, constantly on high alert, start releasing more inflammatory cytokines (like IL-6 and TNF-α). These signals trigger the production of C-reactive protein (CRP) in your liver – a key marker we often test for when assessing inflammation levels. Your body's alarm system becomes stuck in a feedback loop, each component amplifying the others.

Modern life doesn't help. Poor sleep disrupts your circadian rhythm, affecting the production of anti-inflammatory compounds; processed foods, high in advanced glycation end-products (AGEs), trigger inflammatory responses; chronic stress pumps out cortisol, which can dysregulate your immune system. Environmental toxins, sedentary lifestyles and even social isolation all contribute to this inflammatory burden.

Think of it like this: your body's inflammation response was designed for a world of acute physical threats – infections, injuries, predators – but now it's dealing with chronic, low-grade threats it never evolved to handle. Imagine having a state-of-the-art security system that's triggered by Wi-Fi signals – the response is real, but it's not quite fit for purpose.

The Cellular Players.
At the heart of both acute and chronic inflammation are your immune cells, each playing a unique role:

Neutrophils are your rapid response team, arriving first at the scene of injury or infection.

Macrophages follow, engulfing pathogens and damaged cells, while releasing cytokines to coordinate further immune responses.

T-cells and B-cells provide targeted responses, remembering specific threats for future encounters.

But in chronic inflammation, this well-choreographed dance becomes a chaotic mosh pit. These immune cells start producing excess inflammatory mediators, leading to tissue damage and accelerated ageing. The very system designed to protect you begins to cause you harm.

The Path Forward.

Understanding this distinction between acute and chronic inflammation isn't just academic; it's revolutionary for how we approach health and ageing. While acute inflammation is your friend, helping you heal and fight off invaders, chronic inflammation is the silent troublemaker behind everything from accelerated ageing to major health concerns.

But here's the empowering part: once you understand this cellular soap opera, you can start directing the show. Every lifestyle choice, from what you eat to how you sleep, can help restore balance to your body's inflammatory response. It's about turning your internal SWAT team from an overzealous force into a well-regulated, efficient unit that knows exactly when to spring into action – and when to stand down.

As we race forward in time, the way we think about ageing is changing. Scientists are digging deeper – literally – beneath the skin's surface to uncover the secrets of ageing at a cellular level. Remember when 'anti-ageing' was all about looking younger? Well, there's been a revolution, and it's about time! It isn't just about chasing the fountain of youth or erasing wrinkles anymore, it's about cracking the code of how our bodies age and finding ways to give those processes a nudge in the right direction; the goal has shifted from simply adding years to life to adding life to those years. Think about it – what's the point of living to 100 if you can't enjoy the extra decades? People want to reach their twilight years with energy, with mental clarity and, yes, looking their best.

This new concept is called your 'health span' – the period of life spent in good health, free from chronic diseases and debilitating conditions. And guess what? Your skin plays a starring role in this story. Think of it as solving a complex puzzle where each piece represents a different aspect of ageing: cellular health, DNA repair, inflammation and metabolic processes. This really isn't about vanity; it's about maintaining vitality throughout our extended lifespans. Modern research focuses on interventions that could help us achieve the trifecta of longevity, health and appearance. And the exciting part? Many of the same factors that keep your skin healthy – like protection from UV damage, good nutrition, stress management and adequate sleep – also contribute to your overall health span.

Your skin is your body's early warning system for ageing; when we see premature ageing in the skin, it often reflects what's happening inside the body. It's like when your phone's screen starts glitching – it usually means there's an internal issue that needs attention. While we once viewed eczema and psoriasis as purely surface-level concerns, groundbreaking research has revealed them as warning signals from within. Studies show that people with these conditions face significantly higher risks of heart problems – a discovery that has revolutionised our understanding of skin inflammation.

This is why the latest approaches to skin health are about supporting your skin's fundamental health in ways that benefit your entire body. For example, the same collagen degradation that causes sagging skin also affects your joints and blood vessels. The inflammation that shows up as redness or breakouts on your face might signal systemic inflammation affecting your internal organs. By taking care of your skin, through evidence-based treatments and lifestyle choices, you're not just investing in your appearance, you're simultaneously supporting your body's longevity pathways and contributing to your overall health span.

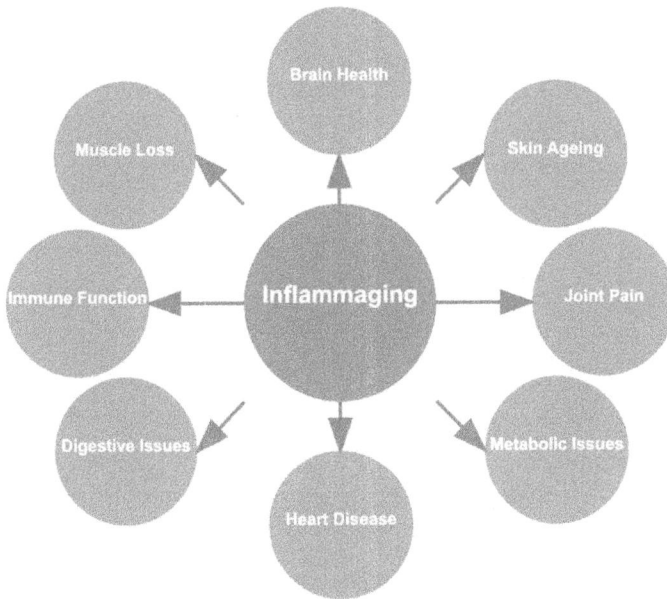

The impact of Inflammaging

Let's get real here, when you look in the mirror and feel great about what you see, it impacts everything from your confidence to your willingness to stay socially active. (And social connection? That's one of the biggest predictors of a long, healthy life. See how it all connects?) This holistic approach to ageing marks an exciting new frontier where beauty, health and longevity come together. Think of it like a Venn diagram from school, with ageing sitting right in the centre, connecting it all.

Twenty years ago, researchers began exploring this phenomenon, which they termed 'inflammageing'. And today, it is the latest buzzword in the science of ageing. Ageing is inevitable and, I believe, a gift, but *how* we age is increasingly within our control. The goal isn't to stop time, it's to help you thrive throughout your entire life journey, with skin that reflects the vitality you feel inside. And when it comes to ageing well, understanding and managing inflammation isn't just one piece of the puzzle – it's the foundation everything else builds upon.

PART ONE:

The Core Ageing Blueprint

CHAPTER 1:
THE SKIN EDIT

It's All About Your Skin

I have some bad news for you: your skin's ageing process began long before you ever noticed your first wrinkle.

As we get older, our skin becomes the canvas that tells the story of our experiences – from those carefree days spent lying in the sun smothered in SPF-0 during our twenties to the stress of sleepless nights fuelled by 'grown-up stuff' with deadlines and responsibilities. Your skin is a remarkable organ, serving not only as a protective barrier but also as an outward reflection of your inner health and wellbeing, and understanding it goes far beyond managing visible ageing – it's about recognising your body's most brutally honest whistleblower.

Ever found yourself completely stressed about an important presentation, only to wake up looking less like the glowing goddess you aspire to be and more like a pizza? Been there! Those late-night kebabs and the missed and looming work deadlines don't just disappear into the void, they show up uninvited as breakouts, dullness and dehydration. Those dark circles aren't just crying out for a better eye cream, they're telling tales about your Netflix binge-watching habits. Here's the scientific truth we've witnessed over decades of clinical experience: your skin is unabashed about how you're living your life. When we see these signs, we're not just seeing surface issues, we're seeing a clear reflection of daily habits and stressors. By understanding this intimate connection between lifestyle and skin health, we can make informed choices that support both our skin's vitality and overall wellbeing for years to come. After all, your skin isn't just being dramatic – it's being honest!

Let's get real about what 'nurturing our skin' actually means because, yes, it can sound a bit 'waffly'! When we talk about 'self-care', we're not suggesting you need to spend hours meditating in a candlelit bath (though, if that's your thing, go for it!); we're talking about practical, science-backed habits that make a real difference. It's about understanding that your morning cortisol spike can trigger oil production, so maybe that high-stakes meeting needs strategic skincare prep. It's about knowing that your skin's repair mechanisms work hardest between 10 p.m. and 2 a.m., so those Netflix binges might be costing you more than just sleep. And those 'mindful choices' about products? (That's code for 'stop throwing money at every trending ingredient on Tik-Tok.') Your skin needs consistency, not the latest viral sensation. Nurturing your skin is about building a routine that works with your skin's natural processes, not against them.

Have you ever wondered why that expensive serum isn't giving you the promised 'instant results', or why that pimple seems to take forever to go? To understand, we need to dive beneath the surface – let's go back to basics and look at skin anatomy, because understanding your skin's architecture is the key to transforming it.

Anatomy of the Skin.
Your skin is far more than a protective covering; it's your body's largest organ. For the data crunchers amongst you, the average woman's skin has a surface area of around 16,000 cm², and its complexity never ceases to amaze me. Daily, I see how this incredible system adapts, heals and responds to the insults we throw at it.

Let's start by uncovering the fascinating structure of skin – a dynamic organ composed of three distinct layers, each with a crucial role in protecting, supporting and enhancing your overall health and appearance.

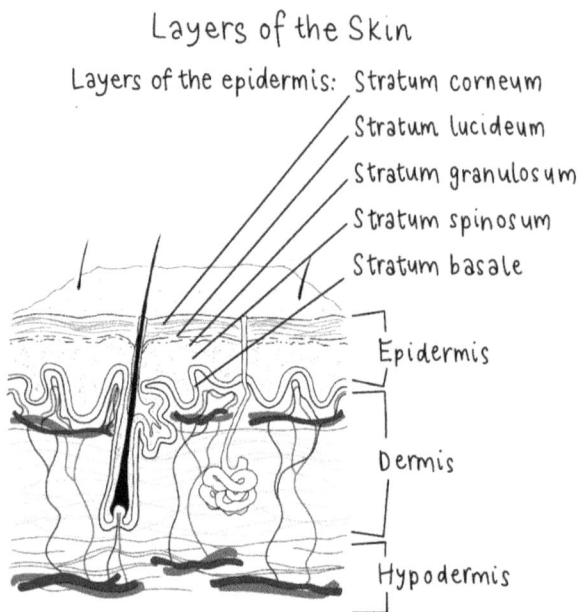

The Skin Anatomy

The Top Layer: The Epidermis.

The epidermis, your outer layer, acts as your body's frontline; it's here that the daily drama of protection and renewal plays out. The main resident cells are called keratinocytes. Their journey begins in the epidermis's basement level (*stratum basale*) where fresh, plump cells are born. These young keratinocytes are full of life and actively dividing.

As they move up, these cells begin to change. In the next level (*stratum spinosum*), they become more polygonal and develop strong connections with their neighbours, like building bridges between houses. Here, you'll also find special cells called Langerhans cells, keeping watch for any unwanted intruders.

Moving higher up (*stratum granulosum*), the keratinocytes start to flatten out and fill with tiny granules, basically packing their bags with special proteins called keratin, getting ready for their final transformation.

Finally, reaching the top layer (*stratum corneum*), the keratinocytes are now completely flat and filled with tough keratin, like tiles on a roof. They form your skin's waterproof barrier, a protective shield that keeps moisture in and harmful things out. Eventually, they naturally shed off, making way for new cells from below.

This entire journey, from birth to shedding, takes about four weeks and is a carefully orchestrated and constant cycle of renewal that keeps your skin healthy and strong.

The Middle Layer: The Dermis.

The dermis, your skin's middle layer, holds the essence of your skin's vitality – like the services and utilities of your skin city.

Here you'll find all the goodies like collagen and elastin, the proteins responsible for your skin's strength and bounce. Collagen and elastin fibres weave throughout the dermis like a complex tapestry: collagen acting like sturdy rope, giving your skin its strength and structure; elastin like tiny rubber bands, letting your skin stretch and bounce back when you move. Together, they create a flexible but strong network that keeps your skin resilient and youthful.

Tiny blood vessels weave through the dermis, like a miniature irrigation system, delivering essential nutrients and oxygen to feed the skin cells and take away waste products. They're also why you blush when embarrassed or turn pale when scared, and they expand or contract to help regulate your body temperature.

Scattered throughout are hair follicles. Each follicle has its own sebaceous (oil) gland, producing a natural moisturiser to keep your skin and hair healthy. Nearby, sweat glands work like tiny sprinklers, helping to cool you down when you're hot.

Perhaps most remarkably, the dermis houses an intricate network of nerve endings. These are tiny sensors, each specialising in different sensations. Some detect pressure, others respond to temperature, and some react to pain. They are why you can feel the lightest brush of a feather or know instantly when something's too hot.

All these components work in harmony, making the dermis not just a layer of skin but a dynamic, living community that keeps your skin healthy, responsive and alive.

The Fatty Layer: The Subcutaneous Tissue/Hypodermis.

The next layer down is the subcutaneous tissue, which sits beneath the outer layers of your skin, playing a vital yet frequently neglected role in its anatomy. This deepest layer serves multiple functions: it stores energy, provides insulation and contributes to the youthful volume of your face.

As we age, alterations in this layer play a significant role in the visible signs of ageing, especially the loss of facial contours and skin firmness. It is this very layer that occupies much of my time in the clinic as I work to replenish lost volume and restore youthful appearance. So, I'm an avid fan of this layer.

As your skin ages, it becomes increasingly vulnerable to dehydration and environmental damage. The production of natural moisturising factors declines, and the skin barrier becomes less effective at retaining moisture. These changes do not happen uniformly; certain areas of your skin may show signs of ageing sooner than others, influenced by genetics and environmental exposure.

Understanding your skin's structure and function provides the foundation for making informed choices about its care. Your skin is far more than a simple barrier; it's a complex, living organ that adapts and responds to both internal and external changes. From its protective outer layer to its deepest cushioning tissues, each part of your skin plays a vital role in maintaining your health and appearance.

Internal Factors.

Your skin's renewal process is quite complex, and the ageing process affects different areas of your face in distinct ways. You might notice your cheeks losing volume while your jawline is becoming saggy. These changes reflect the complex interplay between bone structure, fat distribution and skin elasticity. Understanding these patterns helps explain why effective anti-ageing strategies often require a multi-pronged approach.

In youth, fresh cells replace old ones every four weeks, maintaining a healthy, vibrant appearance. However, this process gradually slows as we age, beginning in our late teens and becoming more noticeable by our fifties, which affects not just appearance but also the skin's ability to heal and protect itself. It's depressing news, isn't it?

The subcutaneous layer gradually diminishes, leading to changes in facial contours, the appearance of fine lines and wrinkles, folds and jowls, i.e., the effects of gravity.

Hormonal changes, too, significantly influence your skin's behaviour. During adolescence, increased hormone levels can boost oil production, leading to breakouts; women often notice skin changes during their monthly cycle, pregnancy and menopause; and after menopause, declining oestrogen levels can accelerate the breakdown of collagen, making skin care strategies even more important.

Understanding these changes helps explain why your skin needs different care at different life stages. Young skin, like a fresh elastic band, snaps back quickly no matter how much you stretch it. In our twenties, it is resilient and forgiving, bouncing back readily from late nights or forgotten sunscreen. The repair processes work overtime, efficiently maintaining that healthy glow.

As we move through our thirties and into our forties, our skin starts telling a different story. That elastic band has been stretched too many times; it's still functional but not quite as springy. The natural production of collagen and elastin begins to slow, making skin less quick to recover, and the barrier function needs more support to keep moisture locked in and environmental stressors out.

By our fifties, these changes become more visible on the surface. It's like our skin's 'bounce-back team' is working with reduced staff! The scaffolding of collagen and elastin, which kept everything tight and firm in our youth, isn't as robust.

Even with access to the best skincare technology and treatments, our skin behaves differently from what it did decades ago.

But this isn't about fighting a losing battle with time; it's about understanding and supporting our skin's changing needs. Just as we adjust our diet and exercise as we age, our skin care should evolve, too. The goal is to work with our skin's natural processes, not against them, helping it function at its best at every age.

External Factors.

On top of these biological facts, environmental factors also play a significant role in your skin's health. Modern life brings with it pollution, stress and lifestyle choices that all leave their mark on our skin. Supporting your skin's health requires understanding these daily challenges – from UV radiation to air pollution, from central heating to air conditioning. Each one can affect your skin's ability to maintain its protective barrier and renewal processes.

Sunshine.

While UV radiation stimulates vitamin D production, essential for bone health and immune function, it's also the primary cause of premature ageing and can damage skin cell DNA. Though, let's be honest, those of us in less sun-blessed locations could probably use a little more natural glow!

While our friends in tropical paradises are diligently seeking shade from their year-round sunshine (we're looking at you, Australia), many of us in cloudier climates are playing a complicated game of 'catch enough rays without catching too many rays'. It's quite the paradox: trying to get sufficient vitamin D while also protecting our skin from sun damage. With all the UK's grey skies and drizzle, we might need to consider a sun lamp as a staple in our skincare arsenal. Though, perhaps we shouldn't complain too much, at least we're not having to check for spiders before starting our skincare routine!

Sun damage isn't always immediately visible – like a bank account with regular, small withdrawals, the effect accumulates over time, often becoming apparent years later. However, the visible signs of ageing often first appear in areas most exposed to the sun; it's common to see a youthful face paired with an aged neck, often due to neglecting the décolletage when applying SPF, as well as the skin being thinner and having less fat for cushioning. Your sun-damaged skin may become more translucent, revealing the delicate network of blood vessels beneath; it might develop an uneven tone, with both pigmented and non-pigmented patches creating a distinctive pattern.

Diet.
The connection between diet and skin health becomes more apparent as we age. Your skin requires specific nutrients to function optimally – proteins for repair, healthy fats for barrier function, and antioxidants for protection against environmental damage. A balanced diet rich in these nutrients provides your skin with the building blocks it needs for repair and renewal.

Hydration also plays a crucial role in skin health, but it's more complex than simply drinking water. Your skin's ability to retain moisture depends on its barrier function and the presence of natural moisturising factors. As we age, both mechanisms become less efficient, making proper skincare increasingly important.

Modern research has revealed fascinating insights into skin health. We now understand that skin doesn't just protect us physically, it responds to stress, reflects our internal health and even influences our emotional wellbeing. This connection between skin health and overall wellness becomes more apparent with each new scientific discovery.

In my clinical practice, I've observed how lifestyle choices profoundly impact the health of the skin. Smoking, for instance, doesn't just stain your fingers and give you smelly breath, it literally doubles the rate at which your skin breaks down collagen and elastin. Scary fact! And once damaged, these essential proteins are not easily replaced.

Did you know your skin's function changes throughout the day and night? During daylight hours, it focuses on protection: defending against UV radiation, pollution and other environmental challenges. At night, it shifts into repair mode, with cell renewal and regeneration reaching their peak during the early hours of sleep. Understanding this rhythm helps explain why good sleep isn't just about feeling refreshed, it's fundamental to your skin health.

Your skin also hosts millions of beneficial bacteria that form part of your skin's microbiome. This delicate ecosystem helps maintain skin health by competing with harmful organisms and supporting your skin's immune function. Modern lifestyle factors, including over-cleansing and antibiotic use, can disrupt this balance.

Your skin is unique to you, influenced by your genetics, lifestyle and environmental factors. While we can't stop the ageing process, understanding how your skin functions will help you make better choices about its care and protection.

#DrVixTakeaways

1. Your skin is your body's most honest whistleblower – it visibly reflects your lifestyle choices, stress levels and overall health long before other symptoms appear. Those late nights and missed meals don't just disappear, they show up as breakouts, dullness and dehydration.

2. Your skin has three critical layers: the protective epidermis (outer layer), the collagen-rich dermis (middle layer), and the volumising subcutaneous tissue (bottom layer). Each plays a vital role in keeping your skin healthy and youthful.

3. The skin's renewal process naturally slows as we age – while young skin replaces cells every four weeks, this process becomes less efficient in our late teens and is notably slower by our fifties.

4. Your skin functions differently during the day and the night – it focuses on protection during daylight hours and switches to repair mode at night, with peak regeneration occurring during early sleep.

5. Environmental factors, especially UV exposure, significantly impact skin ageing – even in less sunny climates. Finding the right balance between getting enough vitamin D and protecting against sun damage is crucial for skin health.

CHAPTER 2:
YOUR INTRINSIC AGEING SOFTWARE

Decoding the Programme You Were Born With

Have you ever wondered at one of nature's most intriguing paradoxes: identical genetic blueprints expressing ageing in very different ways? Within families, particularly among siblings, the differences become strikingly apparent. One sister may retain youthful vitality well into her fifties, while another shows pronounced signs of ageing decades earlier. Even more fascinating is how your own face ages asymmetrically, with certain areas betraying time's passage before others.

Intrinsic ageing also helps explain why people from different ethnic backgrounds tend to age at different rates. For example, individuals with more melanin in their skin often have a natural layer of protection against UV damage, which can delay the formation of fine lines and pigmentation issues. This means that anti-ageing treatments may work differently across ethnicities, as each skin type has its unique structure and ageing timeline.

Intrinsic ageing is like your body's built-in operating system – pre-programmed and running quietly in the background, whether you're aware of it or not. It's your biological clock, ticking steadily to a rhythm set by your DNA long before you were born, like an internal hourglass that measures time, not in sand but in cellular changes, hormonal shifts and subtle biological transformations. In short, you can thank (or blame) your parents for it!

While we often focus on external factors like sun damage, smoking and pollution (we'll get to these later), this chapter delves into these preset ageing patterns encoded in your genes, which tick away regardless of environmental factors. While we can't rewrite this genetic code, understanding these internal age-ing mechanisms isn't just about satisfying scientific curiosity, it's about recognising which aspects of ageing we can influence and which we need to work with rather than fight against.

So, brace yourself for an insight into the Twelve Pillars of Ageing, the master controllers of how we age. This isn't just any scientific theory; it's the hottest topic shaking up the longevity world right now and, in clinic, understanding these fundamental processes has revolutionised how we approach ageing and given us powerful tools to influence the ageing process.

Think of these pillars as the secret code that determines whether you'll age like a fine wine or ... well, you get the picture. Some of them might sound intimidatingly scientific, but don't worry, I'll break down each one into understandable concepts that reveal how they affect your daily life and, more important-ly, what you can do about them. Are you ready to discover what makes your biological clock tick?

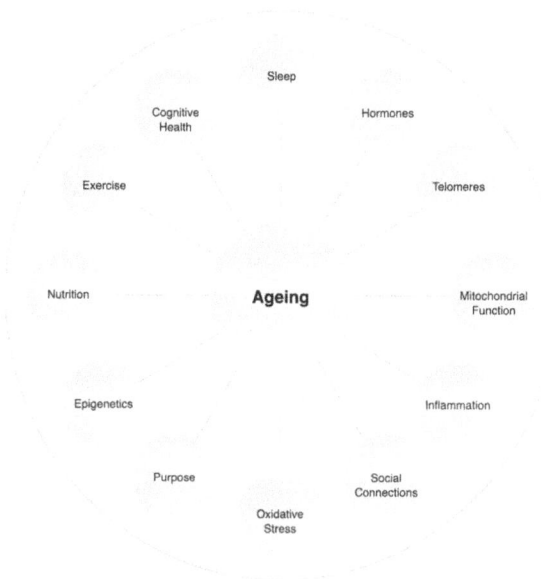

The Twelve Pillars of Ageing

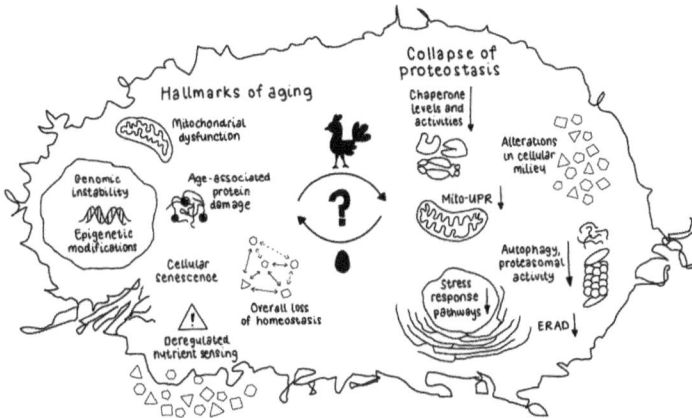

The Hallmarks of Ageing

The Twelve Pillars of Ageing.

From the Twelve Pillars, six are considered *intrinsic* ageing factors, and it is these we are going to study more closely here.

Pillar 1: DNA Damage – Your Genetic Blueprint Under Siege.

As we age, our DNA faces an ongoing barrage of challenges. Your genetic code is like an ancient manuscript – over time, words get smudged, pages tear, some information becomes harder to read and free radicals, like unwelcome editors, create random changes to the text. While your cells have built-in proofreaders (DNA repair enzymes), they become less efficient with age, like having fewer and fewer skilled restoration experts available to fix the damage. These accumulated mutations lead to cellular dysfunction, affecting everything from collagen production to skin barrier function.

We talked about why some people seem to age more 'gracefully' than others, even within the same family. Why is this? The answer lies in tiny structures called telomeres, your body's biological timekeepers. You may not have even heard of them, but don't worry; I find telomeres fascinating because they offer tangible insights into not just why we age, but how we might influence that process.

First, let's understand where we can find them. Inside nearly every cell in your body, you'll find your DNA – essentially your personal instruction manual containing about 20,000 genes that determine everything from your eye colour to how efficiently you process nutrients. This DNA is carefully packaged into structures called chromosomes, rather like how a long string can be wound around a spool to keep it organised. And at the ends of each chromosome, you'll find your telomeres – protective caps made up of repeated DNA sequences (TTAGGG in humans, if you're curious about the specifics).

Humans typically have 46 chromosomes, arranged in 23 pairs. These pairs are like the volumes of an encyclopaedia set, each containing specific chapters of information about how to build and maintain your body. During most of your life, your cells are constantly dividing to replace old or damaged tissue, and each time this happens, all this genetic information needs to be copied accurately. While the shoelace aglet analogy is commonly used, I prefer to think of telomeres as the protective plastic coating on the ends of electrical wires. Without this coating, the wires would fray and potentially cause short circuits. Similarly, without telomeres, our chromosomes would become damaged, compromising our cells' genetic information and sending out dodgy messages.

Here's where it gets interesting – and problematic. Every time a cell divides, the DNA copying 'machinery' can't quite reach the very end of the chromosome, rather like trying to photocopy a document while part of it is stuck under the copier's edge – you lose a tiny bit of information each time. Nature's solution to this 'end replication problem' is brilliant: telomeres serve as a disposable buffer zone. Every time a cell divides, it's the telomeres that get shortened not the crucial genetic information inside the chromosome. So, they act as expendable sections at the end of each chromosome that can be sacrificed without losing anything important.

Initially, at birth, our telomeres are around 10,000 base pairs long (think of base pairs as the individual letters in your genetic alphabet). With each cell division, we lose anywhere from 30 to

200 base pairs from our telomeres. When telomeres reach a critical length – around 4,000 base pairs – cells typically stop dividing through a process called senescence.

This cellular countdown serves multiple essential purposes, each critical to maintaining our health. First, it stops unlimited cell division. This is important; it means our cells are programmed to stop dividing after a certain point, which is a protective mechanism. If cells could divide indefinitely, they would risk accumulating mutations over time, potentially leading to cancer. By setting a natural limit, the chances of uncontrolled growth are reduced, safeguarding against the formation of tumours. Also, as cells reach the end of their lifespan, they send signals to indicate they're ageing and should be replaced. This prompts the body to activate its repair systems, encouraging new, healthy cells to take over. This turnover helps maintain youthful, functional tissues, ensuring that old or damaged cells don't linger, which would otherwise lead to tissue deterioration. Together, these mechanisms form a finely tuned system that balances cellular renewal with protection, helping to preserve our health as we age.

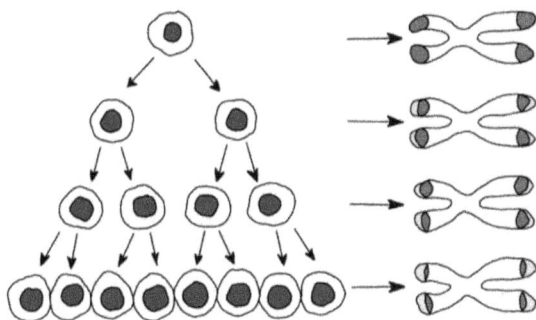

Cell division and Telomere Shortening

So, basically, this telomere countdown acts like a quality-control checkpoint within our tissues, ensuring that only healthy, viable cells continue to function and filtering out older cells. By doing so, the body maintains the structural integrity and efficiency of its organs, skin and other tissues, ultimately promoting overall wellbeing.

The Telomerase Twist.

No, this isn't a new, funky cocktail. Nature has provided an interesting plot twist in this story: an enzyme called telomerase, which can rebuild telomeres.

(Enzymes are specialised proteins that speed up vital chemical reactions. Like a lock and key, each enzyme has a unique shape designed to work with specific molecules, transforming them into something your body needs. Without these tireless workers, even basic processes like digestion would grind to a halt.)

Certain cells in your body, like reproductive and stem cells, produce telomerase to maintain their telomeres' length. However, most adult cells produce little or no telomerase – and for good reason. While it might seem ideal to keep all our telomeres long forever, unlimited cell division, as we said, could lead to cancer.

One fascinating aspect of telomeres is that they don't shorten at the same rate in everyone; like different brands of candles, some burn faster than others. Your telomere shortening rate is influenced by both genetic factors (which brand of candle you bought) and lifestyle factors (how often you burn that candle). For someone interested in knowing their biological age, a simple finger-prick blood test can now provide telomere analysis. The result typically includes your average telomere length compared to others your age along with an estimate of your biological age.

However, what's most valuable isn't a single measurement but tracking changes over time, like having a biological pedometer counting down your cellular age rather than your steps. These measurements can reveal if you're ageing faster or slower than average for your age group. However, I always emphasise that a telomere test isn't a crystal ball; it's more like a snapshot of your cellular health at a moment in time, which can help guide life-style interventions.

You may be asking yourself why this is relevant. What do short telomeres actually mean? Through years of research and clinical observation, scientists discovered that telomere length correlates with various health conditions. (Interestingly, people with shorter telomeres have up to three times higher risk of heart disease) Also, short telomeres can significantly impact your immune system's effectiveness. I often explain to patients how ageing immune cells with shortened telomeres are like tired soldiers – less efficient at fighting off infections and managing inflammation.

But why are they relevant to your skin health and the ageing process? It is your skin cells that are particularly vulnerable to telomere shortening because they're constantly renewing. When telomeres become too short, collagen production decreases, skin cell renewal slows down, healing capacity shrinks and those fine lines and wrinkles appear more readily.

So, we are going back to your lifestyle factors, the good, the bad and the ugly.

What Shortens Your Telomeres?
Let's talk about what's eating away at your cellular timekeepers. Telomeres, those protective caps on your chromosomes, face constant threats in our modern world. They are the canaries in your cellular coal mine – often the first to show signs of stress and environmental damage.

1. Stress: The Silent Telomere Thief.

   The impact of chronic stress on your telomeres is startling; every time your cortisol levels spike, they suffer. Research shows that every major life stressor might age your cells by an extra year. That demanding job, those sleepless nights worrying about deadlines; they're literally shortening your cellular lifespan.

2. Sleep: Your Telomeres' Best Friend.

   Quality sleep isn't just about feeling refreshed, it's essential for telomere maintenance. Getting fewer than six hours of sleep correlates with shorter telomeres, while disrupted sleep patterns interfere with cellular repair mechanisms. It's like trying to repair a building without giving the construction crew enough time to work.

3. Environmental Assaults.

    From air pollution to UV radiation, environmental toxins also wage war on your telomeres. Smoking is particularly damaging, attacking telomere length through multiple pathways. Think of these environmental factors as constant erosive forces wearing away at your cellular protection.

#ActionableSteps

Here's where things get exciting; the good news is there are ways of protecting your telomeres. While we can't stop them from shortening entirely, we have more control over the rate of decline than previously thought. Every lifestyle choice you make either protects or challenges these crucial cellular timekeepers.

1. Exercise: Your Cellular Youth Potion.

    Regular exercise, particularly moderate aerobic activity for 30–40 minutes daily, can reduce telomere shortening by up to 24%. High Intensity Interval Training (HIIT) also shows special promise, while resistance training helps maintain muscle cell telomeres. It's as though working out has a built-in telomere protection program.

2. Nutrition: Feeding Your Telomeres.

    Your diet can either protect or damage your telomeres. Omega-3 fatty acids, especially from wild-caught fish, act like cellular shield boosters. Loading up on antioxidant-rich foods – think colourful berries and leafy greens – provides additional protection. The Mediterranean diet, with its abundance of polyphenols from olive oil, vegetables and, yes, even dark chocolate, also offers particularly good telomere support.

3. The Mindfulness Connection.

   Perhaps most fascinating is how stress management techniques directly impact telomere health. Mindfulness and meditation have been shown to increase telomerase activity; regular yoga, time spent in nature and strong social connections all contribute to telomere preservation.

Pillar 2: The Powerhouse Problem – Mitochondrial Decline.

The next little cellular structures we need to touch on are the mitochondria, your powerplants. These powerhouses are crucial for your skin's vitality, producing the energy that keeps your skin cells functioning optimally.

Mitochondria are fascinating, microscopic structures shaped like tiny kidney beans, varying from 0.5 to 10 micrometres in length. In the skin, you'll find them concentrated in the active basal layer of the epidermis, where cell division is constantly occurring, and abundantly throughout the dermis, especially in fibroblasts (cells that make collagen and elastin to keep your skin strong and stretchy and help repair wounds) where collagen production demands high energy.

Each cell in the body can contain hundreds or even thousands of them, the number of which directly correlates with that cell's energy needs. But here's the interesting part: as we age, or when we're exposed to things like UV radiation and pollution, mitochondria start to decline in both number and efficiency, particularly in areas of high energy demand like the basal layer of your epidermis and in collagen-producing fibroblasts. This energy crisis affects everything from cell turnover to protein production, contributing significantly to visible ageing. Think of it as your skin's batteries gradually losing their charge – when cellular energy declines, everything from repair to renewal slows down. This is why tired, stressed skin often looks dull and lacklustre; it's literally running low on cellular energy.

These remarkable organelles turn the food you eat into usable energy, but they also create free radicals as a by-product, like the exhaust from a car engine. While your body has natural antioxidant systems to handle free radicals, modern life puts extraordinary pressure on these defences. Poor diet, stress, lack of sleep and environmental toxins can overwhelm your mitochondria's protective mechanisms, leading to what scientists call 'oxidative stress'.

Oxidative Stress.

Your genetic code influences every aspect of ageing, from your skin's structural integrity to your natural defence systems. One crucial genetic factor is how well your body manages oxidative stress.

Think of oxidative stress like cellular rust – reactive oxygen species (ROS) gradually corrode your skin's supporting structures from within. This creates a cascade effect within your cells, leading to damaged cellular components, slower repair mechanisms and, eventually, the visible signs of ageing we all recognise.

Recent research has revealed fascinating variations in genes controlling antioxidant enzymes, like superoxide dismutase, which significantly impact how well we manage this oxidative damage.

(Superoxide dismutase is a crucial enzyme that acts as your body's first line of defence against oxidative damage by converting harmful superoxide radicals into less dangerous molecules, helping protect your cells from oxidative stress.)

Oxidative stress isn't just about feeling tired, it damages the very DNA within your mitochondria. When mitochondrial DNA becomes damaged, it produces energy less efficiently and creates more harmful free radicals, accelerating the ageing process at a cellular level. This understanding isn't just academic, it has real implications for how we approach anti-ageing treatments.

What fascinates me most about mitochondrial function is its direct link to visible ageing. When these powerhouses begin to falter, the precision of collagen production drops, cell turnover slows and repair mechanisms become sluggish. It's like watching a city during a power cut – everything slows down, and maintenance tasks start piling up. This relationship is particularly evident in how different areas of our face age. Regions with higher energy demands, like the delicate eye area, often show signs of ageing first. This isn't coincidence, it's a direct reflection of how crucial efficient energy production is to maintaining youthful skin structure and function.

But here's where it gets hopeful: research suggests that mitochondrial function isn't entirely at the mercy of time; certain lifestyle factors can either accelerate or slow their decline. High sugar diets and chronic stress are like throwing sand in these delicate machines, while regular exercise and certain nutrients can help maintain their efficiency. So, we can potentially biohack our mitochondria back to health.

#ActionableSteps

These microscopic timekeepers of our cells tell a story far more complex than simple genetics. While we inherit our initial telomere length from our parents, what happens next lies largely in our hands.

1. Your Diet.

   What you choose to eat profoundly impacts your mitochondrial health. The Mediterranean diet, rich in fish, vegetables, nuts and olive oil, provides key nutrients that support mitochondrial function. Coenzyme Q10, found abundantly in sardines, mackerel and leafy greens, acts like a protective shield for your mitochondria while helping them produce energy more efficiently. Spain, here I come!

2. Your Movement.

   Exercise is one of the most powerful ways to increase mitochondrial function. Physical activity stimulates your cells to create new mitochondria, like adding more powerplants to your cellular cities. This is why regular exercise can make you feel *more* energetic, not less.

3. Your Sleep.

   Sleep quality directly affects mitochondrial health. During deep sleep, your cells repair damaged mitochondria and clear out dysfunctional ones. This is why poor sleep doesn't just make you feel tired, it accelerates cellular ageing.

Understanding how to maintain healthy mitochondria through-out ageing could be key to extending not just lifespan, but health span (the period of life spent in good health). As such, scientists are now exploring ways to enhance mitochondrial function through targeted interventions. This isn't just about living longer, it's about maintaining energy, mental clarity and physical vitality as we age.

For those curious about their cellular age, testing can pro-vide valuable insights. However, these numbers should serve as motivation rather than judgement. They're waypoints on your journey, not destinations.

By supporting mitochondrial health through lifestyle choic-es and targeted supplementation, we can potentially slow the aging process at its cellular source. It isn't about finding a single miracle intervention – it never is. Protecting your telomeres de-mands a comprehensive approach.

#PersonalTale

In practice, I've consistently observed that small, sustainable changes deliver far better results than dramatic lifestyle over-hauls that prove impossible to maintain. Those crash diets, that gym membership – you know what I mean. The beauty of a sustainable approach lies in its compound effects; the same hab-its that support your mitochondria also enhance overall health, from improved sleep quality to better stress resilience.

Your cells respond to every choice you make, each day writ-ing a new page in your ageing story. The path to cellular health begins with sleep. From there, incorporating regular exercise creates a cascade of positive changes that make other healthy choices feel natural rather than forced. Stress management, often overlooked, proves crucial – I've witnessed how chronic stress can unravel even the most diligent health routines.

While we can't halt time's march, we can influence how our cells experience it, making each small, positive choice a deposit in our cellular health bank.

Pillar 3: The Sugar Story – Glycation.

This is the chilling reality about what's happening in your skin right now: sugar molecules are literally sabotaging your collagen and elastin, the proteins that keep your skin bouncy and youthful.

We call this process glycation, and it's as brutal as it sounds. When sugar molecules attack your collagen and elastin, they create advanced glycation end-products (AGEs). These AGEs transform your flexible, resilient collagen into stiff, dysfunctional proteins – akin to taking a brand-new rubber band and leaving it in the sun until it becomes brittle, loses its snap and eventually breaks. The scariest part? This silent damage is happening every day, whether you can see it or not.

Glycation plays a crucial role in intrinsic ageing through the formation of AGEs and their effects on collagen and elastin. We explore this fascinating process in much greater detail in Chapter 7, breaking down how different foods influence the process and what dietary choices can help minimise its ageing effects on your skin.

Pillar 4: The Hormonal Symphony.

Hormones play a critical role in skin ageing, impacting cellular function, barrier health and repair mechanisms. We explore this fascinating topic in much greater detail in Chapter 4. There, we break down the complex interplay between different hormones and your skin's ageing process and explore practical strategies for hormonal skin health.

Pillar 5: Inflammageing – The Slow Burn.

As explained in the opening chapter, inflammageing is when your body maintains a state of chronic, low-grade inflammation, which plays a central role in how our skin ages.

Like having your building's security system stuck on high alert, constantly triggering false alarms that wear down the structure over time, inflammageing is triggered by both internal and external stressors.

Pillar 6: Proteostasis – When Your Skin's Quality Control Fails.

This sounds very complicated, but let me try and simplify your cellular cleanup system.

Your cells constantly manufacture proteins, folding them into precise shapes – kind of like origami at a molecular level. Young, healthy cells have efficient systems, ensuring these proteins fold correctly. However, with age, this process becomes error-prone, leading to mis-folded proteins that can't function properly.

Let's go back to the analogy of your cells being like a busy city with a dedicated cleaning crew. Three main teams work together:

1. **The Repair Team:** Fixes damaged proteins, when possible, like mechanics repairing broken machinery.

2. **The Disposal Squad:** Labels and removes damaged proteins that can't be fixed, like a bin collection service.

3. **The Recycling Unit:** Breaks down larger cellular debris and reuses the parts, like a recycling plant.

As we age, this cleanup crew become less efficient – imagine fewer workers showing up each year. The result? Cellular 'trash' builds up, leading to damaged proteins cluttering your cells, lower-quality collagen and elastin, slower skin repair, more inflammation and an overall decline in cell performance. Unfortunately, this protein chaos contributes to deeper wrinkles, loss of firmness and slower healing – all hallmarks of ageing skin.

Understanding these six of the Twelve Pillars of Ageing helps explain why effective anti-ageing strategies need to be multi-targeted – a holistic approach. No single 'miracle' ingredient can address all these aspects of intrinsic ageing. It needs to be about supporting your skin's natural processes while protecting against further damage.

What fascinates me most is how all these systems are so tightly connected. Your body is a bustling neighbourhood. When the power grid (your mitochondria) starts to flicker, the roads (your blood vessels) might get busier, trying to keep things moving. Meanwhile, the repair crew (your immune system) becomes slower with maintenance, and the communication lines (your hormones) start sending mixed signals. Each system relies on the others to keep the neighbourhood running smoothly, so when one area struggles, the effects ripple throughout.

In clinical practice, understanding these factors is essential for tailoring anti-ageing treatments effectively. When patients come in stressing about wrinkles, I often find myself reminding them how their digestive health, hormone levels and immune function all play crucial roles in their skin's appearance and overall ageing process – they get the full 360° shebang.

Understanding your genetic ageing pattern isn't about accepting fate – it's about being proactive with the right interventions at the right time. Those cellular power stations might be getting tired, but you can support them through targeted nutrition and lifestyle choices. The key isn't fighting your genetics, it's working with your natural timeline while optimising the factors within your control. For instance, someone with a family history of early wrinkling may benefit more from collagen-stimulating treatments, while another individual with naturally thicker skin may require treatments that address elasticity rather than volume loss. Recognising these intrinsic variations allows us to deliver results that are both realistic and customised, helping individuals achieve their best skin at any age.

The secret to managing intrinsic ageing lies in this balance: accepting what nature has programmed while maximising our influence over how that programming plays out. It's about making informed choices that support our skin's health, regardless of our genetic predispositions.

#DrVixTakeaways

1. Intrinsic ageing is your body's pre-programmed software, like a biological clock set by your DNA. While you can't change the code, you can influence how it's expressed through lifestyle choices that support your cellular health.

2. Telomeres act as your cellular timekeepers, shortening with each cell division – and when they wear down, your cells start to show signs of ageing. The good news? Their rate of

shortening can be influenced by lifestyle factors like exercise, nutrition and stress management.

3. Your mitochondria are cellular powerplants that become less efficient with age. When these tiny powerhouses struggle, everything from collagen production to cell repair slows down. But, you can support their function through nutrition, exercise and quality sleep.

4. The six pillars of intrinsic ageing work together like different systems in a neighbourhood. When one system starts to fail, it affects all the others, which is why effective anti-ageing strategies need to target multiple areas.

5. Your genetic code might be fixed, but it's not your destiny. Like a piano, the keys are set, but how you play them creates different tunes. Through targeted interventions and lifestyle choices, you can influence how your genes express themselves and how your skin ages.

CHAPTER 3:
THE AGEING PLOT TWISTS

Extrinsic Ageing: Where Lifestyle Meets Your Lifeline

In our last chapter, we explored your internal ageing software; now, let's tackle the sequel: extrinsic ageing or, as I like to call it, 'everything else that makes you look older than you should'.

If you think of intrinsic ageing as your body's natural narrative, extrinsic ageing is like throwing plot twists into your skin's story. From that 'harmless' sunbathing session in your twenties to last night's wine and Chinese takeaway, every environmental exposure and lifestyle choice leaves its mark, accounting for up to 90% of visible skin ageing. The good news? Unlike your genetic code, these are factors you can actually control.

Understanding the connection between inflammation, skin health and ageing opens new possibilities for intervention. While we can't stop the clock, we can influence how our bodies respond; by addressing inflammation and protecting our skin's barrier function, we might be able to affect not just how we look, but how we age overall.

UV Radiation.
Before we decode the effects of UV radiation, it's important to acknowledge the balancing act: while UV exposure poses risks, it's also essential for vitamin D production – a crucial hormone for bone health, immune function and even skin cell regulation. However, the amount of UV needed for adequate vitamin D is minimal compared to the exposure that causes ageing and damage.

UV radiation affects your skin through three distinct mechanisms, each operating differently but collectively accelerating the ageing process. When explaining this to patients, I compare it to dealing with three different types of damage: one works covertly, causing deep structural changes; another creates immediate visible reactions; while the third remains largely blocked by our atmosphere. Understanding how these three forces work together – not to protect but to age your skin – is crucial for defending your skin's architecture.

Let me introduce you to this troublesome trio and show you how to guard your skin against their different methods of attack.

1. UVA Rays: The Silent Ager.

    These are the undercover agents of skin damage. With longer wavelengths, they reach deep into the skin's dermis, where your precious collagen and elastin are located. While they don't cause the immediate redness of sunburn, they're silently breaking down your skin's structural support. Especially elusive, they're present year-round, penetrating clouds and windows. I often show my patients the famous photo of a truck driver whose window-side face is significantly more aged, vividly illustrating the effects of UVA exposure.

2. UVB Rays: The Sunburn Specialists.

    These are the culprits behind that painful, fiery-red sunburn that can ruin a beach day or your holiday photos. Unlike UVA, UVB rays don't penetrate as deeply, mainly affecting the skin's outermost layers, but they're still dangerous. They directly damage your skin cell DNA, increasing the risk of mutations and, over time, potentially leading to skin cancers.

    Yet, UVB rays do have one redeeming quality: they help trigger the production of vitamin D in your skin, essential for bone health, immune function and even mood regulation. So, short, controlled exposure to sunlight can be beneficial, but without proper protection, the risks of UVB exposure far outweigh the rewards.

3. UVC Rays: The Filtered Friend.

Thanks to our atmosphere, most UVC rays never reach us. The ozone layer is our planetary bodyguard, blocking these potentially harmful rays. However, environmental changes, global warming and the breaking down of the ozone layer mean this protection isn't guaranteed forever.

City Living: The Hidden Aggressor.

Urban living is another unfortunate plot twist in this story. City-dwellers face unique challenges from environmental pollution – ones that most people don't consider when they think about ageing – tiny troublemakers that are invisible but potent. This isn't just about appearances, it's about your skin's fundamental health, and it isn't just an ecological concern making headlines, it's actively accelerating the ageing process of every city-dweller's skin.

I'm fortunate enough to write this from my small coastal town in the New Forest, where our main 'pollutant' might be the occasional gift left behind by the local New Forest ponies. This stark contrast gives me a unique insight into how where we live affects skin health. When I see patients who've moved here from cities, the improvement in their skin's clarity and health after just a few months is remarkable. It's like their skin can finally breathe again.

However, not everyone can escape to the countryside, and understanding how to protect your skin from urban pollution has become increasingly crucial in modern skincare.

When we talk about pollution's effect on skin, we're really discussing a microscopic war zone. Pollution generates free radicals – but what exactly are these? Imagine your skin cells as a perfectly organised house, where every molecule has its proper place and function. Free radicals are like uninvited, drunk party crashers – unstable molecules – who show up and start causing chaos.

For those of you who are more technically minded, free radicals are molecules that are missing an electron (a negative charge), making them desperately unstable. They are like molecular thieves, stealing electrons from healthy cells to stabilise themselves, but unlike regular thieves, who might just take what they want and leave, these molecular burglars create a devastating chain reaction. Each time they steal an electron from a healthy molecule, that molecule becomes a free radical itself, creating a cascade of cellular damage.

Unfortunately, this destruction doesn't just stay superficial. These unstable molecules break into the deeper layers of your skin, damaging crucial proteins like collagen and elastin (the structural beams holding up your skin's architecture). When free radicals attack these support structures, they're essentially weakening your skin's foundation.

But the chaos doesn't stop there. This cellular vandalism triggers your skin's alarm system: inflammation. Your skin calls the skin police to deal with the party crashers, but in doing so, creates even more disruption. This inflammatory response, while necessary, becomes chronic if the assault continues daily, as it does in polluted environments.

So, we now understand that pollution has a double threat: direct cellular damage through free-radical generation and chronic inflammation activation. And the most insidious part? This destruction happens silently and invisibly. You can't feel it happening in the moment, but over time, the cumulative damage appears as premature ageing: wrinkles forming, dark spots appearing and skin losing its resilience and glow earlier than it should.

The Smoking Gun.
While, thankfully, less common today, smoking's effects on skin ageing are worth understanding. Cigarettes cause blood vessels to constrict, reducing oxygen flow, which causes a faster breakdown in collagen; healing becomes compromised; and finally, free-radical damage accelerates.

The good news? (I do like to put a positive spin on most things, and when it comes to smoking and skin health, there's a genuinely exciting silver lining.) Your skin has the extraordinary ability to heal and regenerate once you remove the constant assault of tobacco toxins. It's rather like watching a garden recover after a long drought – given water, the transformation can be remarkable.

#PersonalTale

I've witnessed this regenerative power countless times in clinic. One particularly memorable patient, a 50-year-old who'd smoked for three decades, came to see me about facial rejuvenation. Instead of immediately suggesting treatments, I encouraged her to quit smoking first. Healing in a smoker post aesthetic procedure follows a much slower trajectory than in non-smokers; in addition, they also have a higher complication risk, especially with infection.

When she returned three months later, the changes were striking. The greyish pallor had given way to a healthier glow, those vertical lip lines (what we call 'barcode lines') had softened and her complexion had lost that characteristic dehydrated, leathery texture.

The timeline of skin recovery after quitting smoking is really interesting. Within just 48 hours, your skin's oxygen levels start to normalise. By week two, circulation improves significantly – many patients notice their skin feels less tight and looks less dull. Around the one-month mark, collagen production begins to normalise. And that's when the real magic happens: deep wrinkles start to soften, skin tone becomes more even and that characteristic 'smoker's skin' begins to transform.

In essence, by quitting, you are giving your skin's repair crew the chance to finally do their job properly. When you smoke, it's like having renovators trying to fix a house while someone's actively vandalising it. Stop the vandalism, and suddenly those repair mechanisms can work effectively.

Your Skin's Daily Feast or Famine.

Believe it or not, what you put on your plate has a direct impact on your skin's appearance – and I mean *direct*. That slice of cake or pond-green smoothie isn't just affecting your waistline, it's sending immediate chemical signals to your skin cells, telling them whether to thrive or struggle. Your diet is essentially your skin's instruction manual – every bite either triggers inflammation or helps calm it.

Think of your food choices as text messages to your cells. The sugary snack? It's like sending an 'emergency alert' that triggers inflammation. Whereas the antioxidant-rich salad? It's more like a soothing message, telling your skin cells to repair and rejuvenate. These cellular conversations happen with every single meal, which is why diet is one of the most crucial factors in skin health.

#PersonalTale

I experienced this profound connection firsthand when I started using a continuous glucose monitor to track my blood sugar. Watching how different foods immediately affected my inflammation markers was like having a window into my body's response to everything I ate. That portion of Greek yoghurt and honey that I honestly thought was harmless – my gut response had a very different opinion!

Famine.

The impact of fast-food on your skin and overall health is profound and immediate. For a dramatic illustration of these effects, look no further than the famous *Supersize Me* documentary, where just 30 days of exclusive fast-food consumption led to visible skin deterioration alongside serious health issues.

When you consume highly processed meals – say, a Big Mac, large fries and a large, fizzy drink – your body experiences a cascade of inflammatory responses. Within minutes, a blood sugar spike triggers an insulin surge, while excessive sodium leads to water retention, all of which manifest in your skin as puffiness, breakouts and a dull complexion.

The *Supersize Me* experiment, while extreme, demonstrates how quickly poor dietary choices can impact both our internal health and external appearance. Our modern Western diet reads like a 'most wanted' list for skin ageing; ultra-processed foods, refined sugars and excessive saturated fats aren't just expanding our waistlines, they're triggering internal inflammation that shows up on your face. The skin essentially becomes a mirror, reflecting the chaos happening inside our bodies.

What's particularly interesting is how quickly these changes can appear – sometimes within just days of switching to a high processed-food diet. The good news? Your skin can bounce back when you return to a nutrient-rich, wholefood diet, which acts like your skin's personal bodyguard.

Feast.
1. The Antioxidant Army.

   Eat lots of brightly coloured fruits and vegetables, dark leafy greens, berries and citrus fruits, green tea and dark chocolate (yes, really!). These foods provide the raw materials your skin needs to fight oxidative stress and repair daily damage. They are your skin's construction crew, constantly rebuilding and reinforcing its structure. As the phrase says, 'Eat the rainbow.'

2. Omegas.

   Here's where my passion for test-based nutrition comes in. Through my research, I've discovered that 97% of people have an imbalanced omega-6 to omega-3 ratio. This imbalance is like having too many inflammatory accelerators and not enough brakes. Balancing your omega fatty acids isn't just good for your skin, it's a whole-body approach to managing inflammation and ageing. We go through this in more detail later, in Chapter 8.

3. Hydration.

   Most people think hydration is simply about drinking eight glasses of water a day, but the relationship between hydration and skin health is far more nuanced. Think of your skin's hydration system like a sophisticated irrigation network for a precious garden – it's not just about how much water you pour on, but how effectively that water is distributed and retained.

I don't know about you, but I have multiple 'cool' water bottles to try and encourage me to drink more. Do they work? To be honest, I'm frightful at maintaining my hydration. But the solution isn't just about drinking more water – it's about strategic hydration. And the type of hydration matters too – water-rich foods, electrolyte-balanced drinks and herbal teas all contribute to your body's hydration needs differently.

The timing of your fluid intake matters more than you might think. That 3 p.m. coffee you rely on to get through the afternoon? Caffeine acts as a diuretic (making you pee more), potentially disrupting your hydration balance when your skin's barrier function is most challenged by environmental stressors. And that relaxing glass of wine in the evening? Alcohol is particularly devious; it not only dehydrates you but also triggers inflammation and disrupts your sleep quality, affecting your skin's overnight repair processes.

Your hydration status affects everything from how your cells communicate to how effectively your body removes toxins. Your skin's barrier function acts like a protective seal, preventing moisture from evaporating too quickly – scientists call this trans-epidermal water loss (TEWL). When properly hydrated, this barrier works efficiently, keeping your skin plump and resilient.

#ActionableSteps

So, basically, your daily habits write their story across your face every day – sometimes in ways you might not expect. Let me share what I've learned about how your daily habits shape your skin's future:

1. Sleep: Your Skin's VIP Time for Repair and Renewal.

   Your skin has its own nocturnal maintenance crew. When you fall into deep sleep, something amazing happens: blood flow increases, collagen production kicks into high gear and your skin begins its nightly repair routine. UV damage from that sunny afternoon? Your skin's working on fixing it. Inflammation from stress? Your repair crew's on it. Missing out on quality sleep is like cancelling your skin's essential maintenance appointment – if done repeatedly, eventually, things start to break down.

2. Stress: The Uninvited Guest Who Overstays Their Welcome.

   When you're chronically stressed, your body pumps out cortisol, which isn't your skin's friend. It's like having an overenthusiastic demolition crew in your skin, breaking down collagen, cranking up oil production and compromising your skin's protective barrier. Even wound healing slows down.

I often tell my patients that stress is their skin's annoying neighbour – the less you have to deal with it, the better your skin looks.

3. Exercise: Your Skin's Best Friend.

Every time you get moving, you're giving your skin a mini spa treatment from the inside out, complete with improved collagen production and reduced inflammation. Blood circulation increases, delivering fresh nutrients to your skin cells while whisking away toxins. Even a brisk 30-minute walk can make a difference.

What makes extrinsic ageing both challenging and exciting is that it's largely within our control. Unlike our genetic blueprint, these external factors are like a choose-your-own-adventure book – every choice we make, from what we eat for breakfast to when we go to bed, either deposits into or withdraws from our skin health account.

Looking back at my own journey, from those oil-basted sunbathing days to my current understanding of skin science, I've learned that it's never too late to change your skin's story. Every positive choice – whether it's applying sunscreen, eating an antioxidant-rich meal or getting a good night's sleep – is a step in the right direction. The damage we've done isn't always permanent; our skin has a remarkable ability to heal and regenerate when given the right support. The returns might not be immediate, but they compound over time, much like a well-managed investment portfolio.

The key isn't perfection, it's progress. You don't need to live in a bubble or survive on kale smoothies to have healthy, vibrant skin. (I hate green smoothies; they are just wrong and smell of pond water, IMHO!) It's about making informed choices most of the time and understanding the impact of those choices. Sometimes that glass of wine is worth the withdrawal from your skin health account – the goal is maintaining a healthy balance overall.

#DrVixTakeaways

1. The ageing revolution isn't just about looking younger, it's about extending your health span, the period of life spent in good health. When you invest in your skin health, you're not being vain; you're supporting your body's longevity pathways and overall vitality.

2. Extrinsic ageing factors (those we can control) account for up to 90% of visible skin ageing. From UV exposure and pollution to lifestyle choices and diet, these environmental and behavioural factors are like plot twists in your skin's story that you have the power to edit.

3. UV radiation acts through three distinct pathways: UVA (the silent ager that penetrates deeply), UVB (the sunburn specialist), and UVC (currently blocked by the ozone layer). Understanding this troublesome trio is crucial for protecting your skin's architecture.

4. City living presents unique challenges with pollution-generated free radicals – these molecular thieves steal electrons from healthy cells, creating a destructive chain reaction that accelerates ageing. But the good news? Your skin has remarkable regenerative powers when given the right support.

5. Your daily habits are like deposits and withdrawals from your skin health savings account. Every choice – from that afternoon coffee to your sleep schedule – either supports or challenges your skin health. While perfection isn't necessary, understanding these impacts helps you maintain a healthy balance.

CHAPTER 4:
THE HORMONE HIGHWAY

Your Body's Ageing Signal System

Understanding your hormonal landscape isn't just about managing symptoms, it's about optimising your ageing process. When we recognise how hormones influence everything from collagen production to fat distribution and sleep quality to stress resilience, we can make informed choices that support our body's changing needs. Your hormonal patterns are as unique as you are, but the science that drives them is universal. By understanding these chemical messengers – the architects of ageing – you can take control of how gracefully you age.

In this chapter, we decode the complex interplay between hormones and ageing. We explore how oestrogen affects skin thickness and hydration, why testosterone influences more than just libido and how stress hormones can accelerate ageing at a cellular level. More importantly, we'll discuss practical strategies to support your hormonal health.

You likely think of hormones as those chemicals affecting mood swings or monthly cycles, but they're the hidden architects of ageing, orchestrating far more than your mood swings. Hormones are the unseen conductors of our body's intricate rhythms, controlling everything from energy levels to skin vitality. When it comes to ageing, their influence is immense. These chemical messengers maintain the balance in countless bodily processes, but as we get older, their levels gradually decline, bringing noticeable changes along the way.

In clinic, I regularly see patients frustrated by mysterious skin changes or that stubborn tummy fat that won't budge, completely unaware that hormones are pulling the strings behind the scenes. When these chemical messengers get out of balance, they essentially flip your inflammation switch to permanent 'on' mode. Your thermostat is stuck on high and, eventually, the whole system overheats.

The perimenopause and menopause journey fascinates me, both professionally and personally. (Yes, I've reached that fun stage where I'm now my own case study!) It's like your body's software getting a major update – some systems need to be recalibrated; others require completely new approaches. Yet, many women navigate this transition with outdated information or, worse, no information at all. I've gone from being the doctor explaining symptoms to becoming the doctor experiencing them firsthand – talk about on-the-job training! But this personal insight has only deepened my understanding and passion for helping other women through this transition.

In menopause, it's not just hot flashes. Your collagen production (types I and III) plummets, while matrix metalloproteinases (MMPs) – think of them as molecular scissors that cut up proteins – ramp up, literally breaking down your skin's support structure. MMPs are an overenthusiastic demolition crew, breaking down collagen faster than your body can rebuild it. Elastin caves, too, and suddenly, you're dealing with sagging you never had before. Every time you look in the mirror, something seems a little different, a little less firm.

But it goes deeper. Your facial fat pads start shrinking and sliding south, hollowing out your temples and cheeks. It's why that 'tired look' creeps in, even when you're well-rested. Even your facial bones get in on the act; the maxilla and mandible reshape themselves, weakening your mid-face support and changing your face's fundamental architecture.

It's all connected – a hormonal orchestra that transforms how we age. When your hormones are in balance, every section plays in perfect harmony; but when they're off, the whole symphony falls apart. Understanding this isn't just about vanity, it's crucial for anyone serious about healthy ageing and maintaining their vitality long term. This is why I always tell my patients: treating the surface without addressing hormonal balance is like painting over cracks in a foundation; you might mask the problem temporarily, but you're not solving the underlying issue.

Let's now look at the essential hormones that influence your ageing process.

Oestrogen.

This is perhaps the most fascinating hormone in your ageing story. In your younger years, oestrogen works tirelessly as your skin's natural moisturiser and collagen champion. During peak reproductive years, typically your 20s and early 30s, high oestrogen levels help maintain plump, hydrated skin while keeping inflammation in check throughout your body.

However, as you enter your late 30s, oestrogen levels begin their gradual decline. This subtle shift accelerates during perimenopause, in your 40s and early 50s, before dropping dramatically during menopause. By post-menopause, oestrogen levels can be as much as 60% lower than their peak – and your skin notices this change.

Without oestrogen's protective influence, skin becomes drier and thinner, losing its natural bounce and elasticity. But the changes run deeper than just appearance. As oestrogen levels fall, inflammatory markers throughout your body begin to rise.

So, what's actually happening in the skin? Let's dig into the world of oestrogen receptors, the biological switches that control how oestrogen shapes your skin's health and ageing process:

Oestrogen Receptor Alpha (ERα) manages skin hydration and collagen production, and maintains skin thickness. It's particularly concentrated in facial skin, which is why the face often shows the first signs of oestrogen decline.

Oestrogen Receptor Beta (ERβ) controls inflammation and provides UV protection. These receptors are abundant in dermal fibroblasts, the cells responsible for skin firmness and elasticity.

During perimenopause and menopause, both receptor types become less active as oestrogen levels drop. This decreased activity leads to drier skin, increased inflammation and greater UV sensitivity. The impact is significant – menopausal skin can show up to 30% reduction in collagen content within the first five years of the change.

This creates a double challenge: not only do you have less of the hormone that supports skin health, but you're also dealing with increased inflammation that can accelerate ageing.

The good news? Understanding these hormonal shifts and the different receptor types has transformed our approach to hormonal ageing and skincare interventions; it allows us to be proactive rather than reactive and is why targeted treatments that address both hydration and inflammation are crucial for maintaining skin health during hormonal transitions.

While we can't stop oestrogen's natural decline, we can support our body's ageing process; it's not about fighting these changes, it's about working with your changing chemistry to maintain vitality at every stage.

Progesterone

While oestrogen often steals the spotlight, progesterone deserves an equal say in this hormonal drama. Think of them as a well-rehearsed dance duo – oestrogen is the life of the party (stimulating cell growth), while progesterone acts like the responsible friend who keeps things balanced with its naturally calming, anti-inflammatory effects.

The Oestrogen-Progesterone Balance

During the first half of your menstrual cycle, oestrogen promotes skin cell renewal and that healthy glow. After ovulation, progesterone steps in to balance things out. This hormonal handover explains why many women notice radiant skin mid-cycle, followed by changes before their period.

When progesterone drops dramatically just before menstruation, this withdrawal triggers inflammation, leading to those frustrating pre-menstrual breakouts. While oestrogen keeps oil production in check, progesterone can increase it when out of balance, explaining why skin becomes oilier during the luteal phase.

Beyond Skin: Progesterone's Protective Powers

While we're focusing on skin health, it's worth noting that progesterone's protective effects extend far beyond your complexion. This hormone acts as a guardian for three crucial areas:

Breast Protection: Progesterone helps balance oestrogen's stimulating effects on breast tissue, reducing the risk of excessive cell growth that can lead to breast issues.

Brain Health: Progesterone acts as a natural neuroprotector, supporting cognitive function, mood stability, and sleep quality. Its calming effects on the nervous system explain why many women feel more anxious or experience sleep disruption when progesterone drops.

Bone Strength: While oestrogen gets credit for bone health, progesterone actually stimulates new bone formation. It works alongside oestrogen to maintain bone density, making the decline of both hormones during menopause particularly concerning for skeletal health.

Progesterone vs Progestins: A Crucial Distinction

Natural progesterone has an identical molecular structure to what your ovaries produce, offering gentle, anti-inflammatory effects that support skin barrier function. Synthetic progestins (found in many contraceptives and HRT) are chemically modified and can behave very differently. Some have androgenic properties that increase oil production and worsen acne – explaining why some women's skin deteriorates when starting certain hormonal treatments.

When Balance Goes Wrong

Progesterone Deficiency (often from stress or ageing) creates 'oestrogen dominance', manifesting as increased skin sensitivity, jawline breakouts, and products suddenly causing reactions.

During Menopause, progesterone often drops years before oestrogen, removing its anti-inflammatory protection. Combined with declining oestrogen, this creates accelerated skin ageing, increased sensitivity, and slower healing.

In practice, women who maintain better progesterone levels through lifestyle modifications or appropriate support often have more resilient, less reactive skin with fewer hormonal breakouts. However, hormone balance is highly individual – progesterone isn't just oestrogen's sidekick, it's a starring player in your skin's health story.

Testosterone - It's not just for the men!

While often thought of as a 'male' hormone, testosterone plays a critical role in women's health as well. It is essential for maintaining muscle mass, bone density and skin thickness, all of which contribute to a youthful appearance and physical resilience.

In both men and women, testosterone levels gradually decline with age, which can lead to marked changes in skin elasticity and firmness, and the body's ability to repair itself. As testosterone decreases, the skin becomes thinner and more prone to sagging. This hormonal shift not only affects the way we look but also impacts our strength, energy levels and overall vitality.

Thyroid Hormone.

The often-overlooked thyroid hormone is truly the metabolic maestro of the body, regulating the pace of countless processes that keep us healthy and active. But did you think your thyroid was just about metabolism? Think again. This butterfly-shaped gland plays a crucial role during menopause, often masquerading its symptoms with overlapping hot flashes, mood changes and stubborn weight gain, making diagnosis tricky.

When thyroid hormones are out of balance, your entire body slows down. Energy levels dip, skin repair processes lag and that youthful glow starts to fade. Many patients come to me concerned about 'ageing skin' only to discover that suboptimal thyroid function is the hidden culprit. Low levels result in dull, dry or thinning skin and weight gain, while more severe imbalances can affect hair, nails and even cognitive sharpness.

The thyroid and oestrogen are closely connected, especially in women. As women age and oestrogen levels decline, particularly during menopause, thyroid function can also be affected. Oestrogen plays a role in maintaining the sensitivity of thyroid receptors, which means that lower oestrogen levels can blunt the thyroid's effectiveness in doing its job. This drop in oestrogen can create a feedback loop, where reduced thyroid activity further impacts skin health, metabolism and energy levels. Together, these hormonal changes can accelerate visible signs of ageing, like reduced skin elasticity and increased fatigue.

By understanding the interplay between thyroid and oestrogen, we can better support the body's natural balance and address the root causes of what we often assume are 'just' age-related changes. For some, managing thyroid function alongside hormonal shifts can make a world of difference, revealing that what might look like 'ageing' can be a sign of an underlying imbalance that's worth correcting.

Growth Hormone: The Regenerator.
Growth hormone (GH) is a key player in cellular repair, tissue regeneration and overall vitality. It not only supports the body's ability to heal but also plays a vital role in keeping skin firm, smooth, and resilient, working like an internal repair crew, rejuvenating cells, stimulating collagen production and promoting muscle and bone growth. It's no surprise, then, that the natural decline of GH as we age is often linked to common signs of ageing.

As GH levels start to fall – typically in our 30s and continuing gradually over time – the body's regenerative capabilities begin to slow. This reduction is one reason injuries take longer to heal, muscle mass becomes harder to maintain and skin starts to lose that youthful 'bounce'. And because GH is produced most abundantly during deep and good quality, restorative sleep, getting enough rest becomes essential for maintaining its levels and, by extension, supporting the body's ability to repair itself.

GH is also interconnected with other hormones, including testosterone and oestrogen, which work together to promote tissue health, metabolism and vitality. This complex hormonal orchestra helps explain why lower GH levels can amplify the visible effects of ageing; the decline of one hormone influences others. For example, low GH can contribute to a drop in energy and endurance, making it harder to stay active and leading to a further decrease in muscle tone and skin integrity.

In today's crazy world, where quality sleep is often compromised, maintaining adequate levels of GH can be especially challenging. However, small lifestyle changes like establishing a regular sleep routine, reducing stress and eating a balanced diet can help support natural GH production. Some research even suggests that specific types of exercise, like HIIT and resistance training, may help boost GH levels, offering additional support for tissue repair and overall rejuvenation.

Ultimately, understanding the role of GH can be empowering. It's a reminder that sleep, movement and balanced hormones are not just optional wellness practices but essential aspects of ageing healthfully and maintaining vitality.

DHEA.

Dehydroepiandrosterone – quite the mouthful, so let's stick with DHEA – is often called the 'youth hormone' because of its essential role in maintaining energy, resilience and overall vitality as we age.

I love this hormone! Produced by the adrenal glands, DHEA is a building block to key hormones like testosterone, progesterone and oestrogen, which influence mood, bone density and skin health. It is particularly important for skin health as it supports collagen production, skin hydration and elasticity. It also helps regulate immune function and reduce inflammation, meaning it may help counteract some of the inflammatory processes that accelerate ageing and contribute to chronic health conditions.

Levels of DHEA peak in our twenties and gradually decline with age, and this drop is closely tied to signs of ageing such as reduced energy, decreased muscle mass, thinner, drier skin, a greater susceptibility to wrinkles and even cognitive decline.

In addition to its physical effects, DHEA plays a significant role in mental health and emotional resilience. Research suggests that DHEA may enhance mood, reduce symptoms of depression and improve stress tolerance, partly because it helps buffer the effects of cortisol, the body's primary stress hormone, which can be damaging in high amounts over time. With age, as DHEA levels decline and cortisol levels tend to rise, this imbalance can contribute to the feeling of 'burnout'.

While there's ongoing debate about the effectiveness of DHEA supplementation, some studies have shown that it may help restore vitality and improve quality of life, particularly in those with low baseline levels. However, because DHEA is a potent hormone, it's crucial to approach supplementation carefully and consult a healthcare professional to assess whether it's appropriate.

Understanding DHEA's role gives us valuable insight into how maintaining hormonal balance can support not only our appearance but also our energy, mood and overall resilience as we age. This is why most of my patients receiving Hormone Replacement Therapy (HRT) will be offered this magical 'elixir of youth' hormone.

The hormonal shifts of menopause and andropause represent more than just the end of reproductive years, they're a fundamental reorganisation of your body's chemical communication system. For women, the dramatic drop in oestrogen can trigger a cascade of changes leading to increased inflammation, accelerated collagen loss, changes in fat distribution (especially that middle-aged spread), mood fluctuations and sleep disruption. Men experience their own version, with gradually declining testosterone levels leading to decreased muscle mass, increased body fat, reduced skin thickness and changes in energy and mood.

These hormonal changes don't happen overnight, they send subtle signals long before obvious symptoms appear. The key is learning to recognise these early warning signs. That afternoon energy crash might not just be about your busy schedule, and those new patches of dry skin aren't necessarily just about needing a better moisturiser. In my practice, I've noticed patterns that often indicate hormonal shifts before standard tests show significant changes. Patients frequently report: changes in skin texture and hydration, new areas of stubborn fat despite an unchanged diet, unexplained tiredness, sleep disturbances, mood fluctuations and the classic 'brain fog'.

Here's where modern medicine gives us an advantage; instead of guessing about hormone levels, we can measure them precisely. The key markers I focus on include a comprehensive thyroid panel (not just TSH), oestrogen and progesterone balance, testosterone levels (yes, even in women), cortisol patterns throughout the day, DHEA levels and growth hormone markers. But timing matters. Hormones fluctuate throughout the day and month, so random testing can be misleading.

While HRT can be valuable when properly prescribed, supporting your hormone balance starts with lifestyle choices. Research shows that specific strategies can help optimise your hormonal environment. Sleep becomes increasingly crucial. During deep sleep, your body produces growth hormone and performs cellular repair; poor sleep doesn't just make you tired, it actively disrupts your hormone balance. Exercise affects hormones differently depending on the type and timing. HIIT can boost growth hormone production, while excessive endurance exercise might stress your hormonal system. Nutrition also plays a fundamental role. Certain foods and eating patterns can either support or disrupt hormone balance, and the timing of your meals can be as important as their content.

Modern life presents unique challenges to your hormone balance. Endocrine-disrupting chemicals are everywhere from plastic food containers to personal care products. Understanding and minimising your exposure to these things becomes increasingly important as we age.

Normal vs. Optimal.
Let me challenge something that frustrates me in medicine: the concept of 'normal' test results.

When your blood tests come back marked as 'normal', it reflects a comparison between your results and those of a broad population range, including both healthy and unhealthy individuals. Traditional reference ranges are created by testing a cross-section of the population, including people who are stressed, overweight and generally unwell. Just because your results fall within this range doesn't mean they're ideal for your health. Even more importantly, what's 'normal' for your age might still be far from optimal for vitality and healthy ageing. Think about it – do you want your hormones to be just 'normal' or would you prefer them to be optimal?

The difference between 'normal' and 'optimal' can be profound. I've seen countless patients whose tests were technically normal, yet they felt far from their best. A patient once came to me with severe fatigue, brain fog and premature ageing. Her thyroid tests were all marked 'normal', yet she felt anything but. When we looked closer, her TSH was at the very edge of the reference range. While technically 'normal', it was far from optimal for her body's needs.

Optimal levels are where your body functions best, not just adequately. True optimisation typically means aiming for the upper quartile of the 'normal' range for beneficial hormones and the lower quartile for stress hormones. This is where we see better energy levels, improved skin health, enhanced brain function, a more efficient metabolism and better resilience against stress.

A multipronged approach that aims for 'optimal' addresses the root causes of hormonal imbalances rather than just managing symptoms.

#ActionableSteps

So, what's the solution? Unfortunately, accessing thorough hormone testing and support through the NHS can be challenging due to limited resources and long wait times for GP appointments. In many cases, you may need to consult a private doctor to receive the necessary comprehensive hormone testing and guidance.

Supporting healthy hormone balance requires a multifaceted approach. After decades of experience, I've learned that success lies in the subtleties. It's rarely about dramatic interventions; more often, it's about creating an environment where your hormones can function optimally. In my practice, I've developed a system that integrates regular hormone monitoring, strategic nutritional interventions, targeted supplement protocols, lifestyle modifications and environmental toxin reduction.

Nutrition and Supplement Strategy.
We know that what's on your plate has a powerful impact on your hormones, but this isn't about following some rigid diet, it's about understanding how specific food choices can support your hormone balance naturally.

Cruciferous vegetables like broccoli, cauliflower, kale, cabbage and the dreaded Brussels sprouts, for example, contain compounds that help your body process excess oestrogen, while healthy fats supply the raw materials needed for hormone production.

While nutrition forms the foundation of menopausal wellness, strategic supplementation can provide additional support during this transition. Supporting our bodies with targeted, natural supplements can help manage hormonal fluctuations and their effects.

Magnesium, vitamin D, vitamin B complex and zinc are the key players that form your core support team, helping with sleep, bone health, energy and hormone production.

Diindolylmethane (DIM) is your oestrogen traffic controller. While naturally present in cruciferous vegetables, supplementation can help direct oestrogen metabolism down beneficial pathways rather than potentially harmful ones. This becomes particularly relevant during perimenopause when oestrogen levels fluctuate unpredictably.

N-Acetyl Cysteine (NAC) acts as a precursor to glutathione, your body's master antioxidant. During menopause, when oxidative stress increases, NAC supports your internal detoxification systems and helps maintain cellular health. It's particularly beneficial for skin health and immune function.

Additional targeted support with supplements like Ashwagandha for stress management and sleep and CoQ10 for cellular energy can be added based on individual needs.

Start with the key players, then add others based on your specific needs. Remember, supplements work best alongside a balanced diet and lifestyle – they enhance rather than replace good foundations.

Remember that both supplementation and exercise need personalisation – what works wonderfully for one woman may be ineffective or even counterproductive for another. Morning workouts can help regulate cortisol patterns, and strength training supports growth hormone production, but excessive exercise, particularly in women over 40, can disrupt hormone balance. The key is finding your individual sweet spot in both supplementation and exercise intensity.

When to Seek Professional Support.
Your body sends clear signals when it needs help beyond lifestyle changes.

While feeling tired occasionally is normal during menopause, persistent exhaustion that doesn't improve with better sleep habits and nutrition deserves attention. Watch for clusters of symptoms like unexplained weight fluctuations, significant mood changes, accelerated skin ageing and disrupted sleep patterns that don't respond to your usual strategies. These aren't just inconveniences, they're your body's way of requesting expert intervention.

A healthcare professional can help identify underlying imbalances and create a targeted treatment plan to help you thrive, not just survive, through this transition.

#DrVixTakeaways
1. Your hormones are the conductors of your body's orchestra, influencing everything from skin health to cellular ageing. When they become imbalanced, your inflammation switch gets stuck in the 'on' position, accelerating ageing across all systems.

2. The 'normal' range for hormones isn't necessarily optimal; traditional reference ranges include data from unhealthy populations. Optimal levels – where your body functions best, not just adequately – typically sit in the top quartile of 'normal' for beneficial hormones.

3. Oestrogen isn't just about reproduction, it's also your skin's

natural moisturiser and collagen supporter. DHEA, the 'youth hormone', is equally crucial, supporting both skin health and emotional resilience. Their decline during menopause triggers a cascade of changes affecting everything from skin thickness to fat distribution.

4. Hormonal maintenance occurs between 10 p.m. and 2 a.m. This isn't just about getting enough sleep, it's about aligning with your body's natural hormone production cycles, particularly growth hormone production, which is crucial for repair and regeneration.

5. Supporting hormone health requires a multifaceted approach: proper nutrition (especially cruciferous vegetables for oestrogen metabolism), strategically timed exercise, stress management and, sometimes, medical intervention. One-size-fits-all approaches don't work because your hormonal story is unique.

PART TWO:

The Internal Gut Trilogy

CHAPTER 5:
THE WEIGHT OF INFLAMMATION

More Than Just Numbers on a Scale

Let me paint a slightly different picture of obesity. Your body weight isn't just about numbers on a scale, it's a complex story written in your cells, hormones and inflammation levels. While medical textbooks and the WHO might define obesity as a Body Mass Index (BMI) over 30, or simply as calories in exceeding calories out, the reality is far more nuanced – and fascinating.

Your body is a sophisticated accounting system, but instead of dealing with money, it's balancing energy. When this system gets disrupted – whether through modern processed foods, stress, poor sleep or environmental factors – your metabolic bookkeeper loses control. The result isn't just weight gain, it affects everything from how your cells communicate to how quickly you age.

In clinic, I see how this disruption plays out beyond the obvious. Patients come in concerned about weight, but their bodies are telling a wider story – one of increased inflammation, hormonal chaos and accelerated ageing. This more complex understanding helps explain why the traditional 'eat less, move more' advice often falls short. This isn't just about fitting into smaller clothes, it's about understanding how excess weight fundamentally changes your body's ageing process; we're not just dealing with a simple caloric equation, we're addressing a sophisticated biological system that influences everything from your skin's collagen production to your cellular repair mechanisms.

Obesity is a complex, chronic disease that affects multiple body systems and has far-reaching implications for health and longevity. Beyond the numbers, it is fundamentally a problem of energy regulation where the body's sophisticated weight man-agement systems become disrupted. Like the thermostat in your home that maintains a constant temperature, your body has built-in mechanisms to regulate weight. But various factors can interfere with these systems, leading to progressive weight gain and difficulty losing it.

When we talk about obesity's impact on health, we often think about heart disease, diabetes and joint problems. But there's an-other story unfolding right at the surface – you guessed it – in your skin.

From both clinical practice and a personal perspective, I've observed how excess weight creates a perfect storm of inflam-mation that dramatically affects skin health and ageing. Your fat cells are more than just passive storage units; they're tiny fac-tories, pumping out inflammatory chemicals called cytokines; the more fat cells you have, the more these inflammatory signals multiply. It's like turning up the heat under a pot that's already simmering – eventually, it boils over.

This constant state of inflammation doesn't just affect your internal organs, it creates visible changes in your skin. From ac-celerated ageing and delayed wound healing to increased risk of skin infections and inflammatory conditions, the effects are both profound and far-reaching. So, addressing obesity isn't just about fitting into your favourite jeans, it's about creating an environ-ment where your skin can thrive.

Understanding the relationship between inflammation, obe-sity and the skin is crucial for anyone serious about skin health, whether you're a patient seeking answers or a practitioner devel-oping treatment plans.

The scale of the UK's weight crisis is hard to ignore, and the num-bers paint a striking picture. According to the latest NHS sta-tistics (2021–22), 64% of adults in England are now either over-weight or obese. To break that down, 40.3% of adults have a BMI between 25 and 29.9 (overweight), and 25.9% have a BMI over 30, qualifying as obese. Scary, heh? In the 1970s, only about 40% of adults in England fell into these categories, but that percentage has steadily climbed over the past five decades, with the biggest jumps in the last 20 years.

These numbers aren't just stats, they reflect real-life health impacts, and frankly, they're alarming. According to the UK Government's 2022 Obesity Profile, obesity shortens life expectancy by an average of 3–10 years, obese adults are five times more likely to develop Type 2 diabetes, and weight-related conditions cost the NHS around £6.1 billion each year.

Let's talk money – because the financial impact of obesity is eye-watering. The UK Government's Foresight Report puts the current cost to society at a staggering £27 billion annually. And hold on to your wallets because, if current trends continue, we're looking at nearly £50 billion by 2050. That's not just a number, it's hospitals, healthcare resources and productivity all taking a massive hit.

What's particularly relevant to our discussion – and why these figures matter – is the link between excess weight and inflammation. Let me explain how excess weight fuels inflammation.

Inflammation is a smouldering fire in your body. When you're carrying extra weight, each fat cell acts like kindling, keeping that fire burning. Research shows that people with obesity typically have inflammation levels two to three times higher than those at a healthy weight, measured through a marker called C-reactive protein (CRP). Think of these elevated inflammation levels as smoke spreading throughout your house – it seeps into every room, affecting everything it touches. In your body, this 'smoke' impacts how quickly your skin ages, your heart's health, your joint function, your energy levels and even your brain's performance.

It's a vicious cycle: excess fat triggers inflammation, which makes it harder for your body to regulate weight, which leads to more inflammation. Breaking this cycle isn't just about weight loss – it's about understanding and addressing this hidden fire that's accelerating your ageing process.

Here's what really fascinates me as a skin nerd: the often-overlooked impact of excess weight on your skin's health and appearance. If you're carrying extra weight (specifically, a BMI over 30), you're not just dealing with internal health issues, your skin is fighting its own battles, too. Obesity makes you 40% more likely to develop certain skin infections, your wounds take longer to heal (not ideal if you're considering cosmetic procedures), you're more prone to inflammatory skin conditions (hello, unexpected breakouts and rashes) and – here's the kicker – your skin is literally ageing faster due to those pesky elevated inflammatory markers we talked about earlier.

I see these impacts play out in my clinic every day. Your skin isn't just your largest organ, it's a mirror reflecting your overall health; and when it comes to excess weight, that reflection tells quite a story.

#PersonalTale

Clinical experience has taught me how much excess weight not just affects appearance but fundamentally changes how our bodies heal and fight infection. This isn't about aesthetics or judgement; it's about understanding how inflammation impacts recovery.

One case particularly stands out in which two patients meticulously followed identical post-treatment protocols, yet their healing times were dramatically different. The only significant difference? Their inflammatory status due to weight. While one healed quickly, the other struggled with prolonged recovery.

This pattern appears so consistently that it's changed how I approach treatment planning. Now, I have detailed discussions about inflammation and weight management before proceeding with certain procedures. Understanding these connections helps patients make informed decisions about their treatment journey and sets realistic expectations for recovery.

This kind of real-world evidence reinforces what the research tells us: excess weight isn't just about appearance, every extra pound affects your body's inflammatory status, which in turn influences everything from healing time to treatment outcomes.

Now you have the rather sobering figures, let's look at why this is happening.

Blood Glucose Regulation.

Think of your relationship with food like a banking system. Every calorie is either spent immediately for energy, invested in muscle or stored as fat for future use. But the real story lies in how your body manages glucose (sugar), your cells' primary energy currency.

Your blood glucose regulation is a clever piece of biological engineering. (I remember being able to cite the process by heart back in my med-school days – now I'm not so sure!) However, let's give it a try … When you eat carbohydrates (bread, pasta, etc.), they're broken down into glucose, which triggers your pancreas to release insulin.

(Insulin doesn't work alone. It partners with other hormones like glucagon, which raises blood sugar when it's too low; incretins, which help regulate insulin release; and amylin, which slows gastric emptying. Each hormone plays its part in maintaining balance.)

However, when we continually bombard our system with high-glycaemic foods and excess calories, what should be a finely tuned process and a delicate balance turns into chaos. Your pancreas is put under pressure to produce more and more insulin to manage the flood of glucose. Over time, this constant demand makes your cells resistant to insulin's effects, much like doormen at an overcrowded club refusing entry to guests, no matter how many times they're called. This insulin resistance can lead to a cascade of metabolic problems, increasing the risk of conditions like Type 2 diabetes and contributing to inflammation, which affects everything from your skin to your long-term health.

Taking it back to basics, high-glycaemic foods are those that cause a rapid spike in blood sugar levels after you eat them. The glycaemic index (GI) is a measure that ranks foods based on how quickly they increase blood glucose. Foods with a high GI are quickly digested and absorbed, leading to a sharp rise in blood sugar followed by an equally sharp insulin response. This rollercoaster effect can wreak havoc on your energy levels, appetite control and long-term health.

Here are a few examples of high-GI foods:

- **Refined carbohydrates:** white bread, pastries and most breakfast cereals.

- **Sugary snacks and drinks:** candy, soft drinks and energy drinks.

- **Starchy foods:** white rice, white pasta, potatoes (especially mashed or fried) and cornflakes.

- **Processed foods:** many fast foods, crackers and prepackaged snacks.

High-GI foods are problematic because they cause:

1. **Energy Crashes:** While they provide a quick energy boost, the subsequent blood sugar drop can leave you feeling fatigued, hungry and craving more sugar – a vicious cycle.

2. **Increased Fat Storage:** High insulin levels encourage your body to store excess glucose as fat, often leading to weight gain and visceral fat accumulation (the fat that sits around your organs; I'll explain more shortly), which is linked to inflammation and metabolic diseases.

3. **Chronic Inflammation:** Frequent blood sugar spikes lead to oxidative stress and the activation of inflammatory pathways, affecting not only your metabolism but also your skin, joints and overall health.

4. **Insulin Resistance:** Regularly overloading your system with high-GI foods can desensitise your cells to insulin, increasing the risk of Type 2 diabetes and other metabolic disorders.

5. **Premature Ageing:** High-GI foods accelerate the production of **AGEs**, which damage collagen and elastin in your skin, leading to premature wrinkles and sagging.

Like everything in life, there's a tipping point where insulin resistance turns into inflammation, and this is where things get both fascinating and worrisome. Insulin resistance doesn't just sit quietly in the background, it sets off a chain reaction with far-reaching consequences.

As cells become resistant to insulin, glucose struggles to enter them, leaving your bloodstream with elevated sugar levels. Your hardworking pancreas senses the issue and compensates by producing even more insulin, determined to break through the cellular resistance. But, instead of fixing the problem, this fuels the destructive cycle.

Also, when insulin resistance develops, your body unfortunately becomes extraordinarily efficient at storing fat, particularly around your organs. This is called visceral fat and isn't just passive storage, it's metabolically active tissue that functions like an inflammation-producing factory.

Visceral fat cells (adipocytes) produce their own inflammatory compounds: tumour necrosis factor-alpha (TNF-α), interleukin-6 (IL-6) and various other pro-inflammatory cytokines. These create a state of chronic, low-grade inflammation throughout your body, which create, in effect, a small fire constantly making smoke that damages everything.

High insulin levels don't just manage blood sugar, they act like a switch for inflammation, flipping on multiple harmful pathways:

1. **Direct Inflammatory Signalling:** Insulin stimulates the release of **cytokines** (small proteins that normally help the immune system respond to injury or infection). But elevated insulin turns these mediators into troublemakers, promoting low-grade, chronic inflammation.

2. **Formation of advanced glycation end-products (AGEs):** When excess glucose binds to proteins or lipids, it creates warped, sticky structures called AGEs. These damaged molecules wreak havoc by stiffening tissues, compromising collagen and setting off inflammatory alarms. (We'll dig deeper into AGEs soon – they deserve their own spotlight!)

3. **Oxidative Stress:** High glucose levels generate an overproduction of **free radicals** (unstable molecules that damage cells and tissues). This oxidative stress depletes your body's antioxidant reserves and drives inflammation further, creating a perfect storm for cellular chaos.

The problem with inflammation at this level is that it doesn't stay confined to one area. It spreads its influence, affecting multiple systems and creating a ripple effect throughout the body.

- **Skin Health:** Chronic inflammation weakens your skin's barrier, accelerates ageing and contributes to inflammatory conditions like acne, eczema and psoriasis.

- **Cardiovascular Health:** Inflammatory cytokines can damage blood vessels, increase plaque buildup and heighten the risk of heart disease.

- **Metabolic Dysfunction:** Insulin resistance and chronic inflammation are central players in Type 2 diabetes, making weight loss, energy regulation and metabolic balance even harder to achieve.

- **Gut-Skin Axis Disruption:** Inflammation damages the gut lining, allowing harmful substances to leak into the bloodstream. This not only worsens systemic inflammation but also affects the microbiome, your skin's frontline defence.

Don't worry, there is a silver lining: this tipping point doesn't have to spiral out of control. The secret lies in addressing the root causes of insulin resistance and chronic inflammation, which is about much more than just keeping your blood sugar in check. It's about crafting an environment where your cells can thrive, performing at their best.

Start with balanced nutrition. Think of this as giving your body the fuel it truly deserves. Focus on whole, unprocessed foods, plenty of fibre and low-glycaemic options that help avoid the rollercoaster of sugar spikes and crashes. You don't have to eliminate carbohydrates entirely, it's about choosing lower-GI options that release glucose more gradually and keep you feeling satisfied longer. Some alternatives include: whole grains like quinoa, oats and brown rice; legumes such as lentils, chickpeas and black beans; non-starchy vegetables like leafy greens, broccoli and zucchini; lower-GI fruits such as berries, apples and pears; healthy fats like avocados, olive oil and salmon; and proteins like chicken, turkey, fish and eggs.

Then, take a closer look at stress. Chronic stress doesn't just mess with your mood, it's a major driver of insulin resistance and inflammation; stress hormones can raise blood sugar even when you haven't eaten. Incorporating techniques like mindfulness, yoga or even a brisk daily walk can work wonders to lower cortisol levels and improve insulin sensitivity.

Don't forget about the power of antioxidants. Picture them as tiny bodyguards, neutralising the damage caused by free radicals. Foods like berries, green tea and dark leafy greens are rich in these protective compounds, helping your cells recover and thrive.

Finally, give your body the healthy fats it craves. Omega-3 fatty acids – found in fish, walnuts and flaxseed – are like peacekeepers for your cells, working to counteract the inflammatory pathways stirred up by insulin resistance.

The beauty of all this? By catching the cycle early, you can stop it in its tracks, preventing it from snowballing into more serious, long-term health problems.

So, what does this all have to do with your skin and the ageing process?

Think of your skin, your body's largest organ, as a mirror, reflecting what's happening on the inside. When your blood sugar is poorly controlled and inflammation is running high, your skin takes a direct hit. The constant exposure to inflammatory compounds sets off a chain reaction that affects every aspect of your skin's health and appearance.

Collagen, your skin's support structure, becomes particularly vulnerable. Inflammatory compounds speed up its breakdown while simultaneously making it harder for your body to produce more. It's like having a building where the foundation is being eroded while the construction team is on strike.

Your skin's protective barrier also bears the brunt of inflammatory assault and becomes compromised. The result? Your skin becomes more susceptible to environmental damage, loses moisture more easily and has trouble maintaining its healthy balance.

Hyaluronic acid, your skin's natural moisturiser that gives it that plump, youthful appearance, also takes a hit. Your skin's ability to produce and maintain adequate levels of this crucial molecule decreases, leading to loss of volume and hydration. Rather like deflating a balloon, the surface becomes less smooth and more prone to wrinkles.

But perhaps most concerning is the process of advanced glycation (as mentioned earlier), where, when your blood sugar is consistently high, sugar molecules attach themselves to proteins in your skin. These AGEs accumulate over time, leading to skin that's less elastic, more prone to sagging and shows accelerated signs of ageing.

These changes explain why people with poor blood sugar control often notice their skin ages faster than their years might suggest, their wounds take longer to heal and their skin loses its resilience and glow. It's not just about the number on the scale or even the number on your glucose meter – it's about how these factors collectively impact your skin's ability to maintain and repair itself.

Your blood sugar is like a rollercoaster – the higher the spike, the bigger the crash. The good news is you can transform your health by learning to flatten these curves. After years of treating patients and experiencing my own weight management journey, here's what you really need to know about managing sugar spikes and breaking the inflammation cycle:

#ActionableSteps

Your body's ability to handle sugar changes throughout the day. Just as you're naturally more alert in the morning, your body is better equipped to process carbohydrates earlier in the day. So, use the power of timing and work with your body's natural rhythms.

1. **Front-load your calories:** Your largest meals should align with your body's peak insulin sensitivity in the morning and early afternoon. Big breakfast, small dinner. Also start your day with savoury foods to set you up for the day.

2. **Give your system reset time:** Allow three to four hours between meals for your insulin levels to return to baseline.

3. **Choose smart snacks:** If you need a cheeky snack between meals, choose protein-based options that won't trigger significant blood sugar spikes.

4. *The Movement Solution:* Post-meal exercise is one of the most powerful tools for managing blood sugar. A simple 10-minute walk after eating can reduce post-meal glucose spikes by up to 30%.

#PersonalTale

When I started using my continuous glucose monitor, I was amazed to see how even brief movement changed my blood sugar patterns. The data showed striking differences between days when I remained seated after meals versus those when I took a short walk.

Scientific research backs this up. Movement helps your muscles actively pull glucose from your bloodstream, acting as a natural blood sugar regulator. It's not about intense exercise; even gentle movement can make a significant difference.

The Strategic Order of Eating.

How you eat can be just as important as what you eat. Research shows that simply changing the order in which you consume the foods on your plate can dramatically impact your blood sugar response.

The science behind this is fascinating. Carbohydrates eaten alone/on an empty stomach quickly break down into sugar, causing sharp blood glucose spikes. But when you lead with protein and fibre-rich vegetables, you create a natural barrier that slows this process, turning what could be a spike into a gentle rise. Starting your meal with vegetables (fibre) and then protein and fat before touching carbohydrates can reduce glucose spikes by up to 50%.

#PersonalTale

I learned that my go-to breakfast of yoghurt with honey sent my blood sugar soaring. Then I discovered a game-changing hack: adding pumpkin seeds. These protein and healthy fat-packed seeds transformed my breakfast from a glucose rollercoaster into a gentle wave. Same foods, just a simple addition, yet the impact on my energy levels was remarkable – no more mid-morning crashes, just sustained energy through the day.

Get Some Shut-Eye.

The impact of sleep on blood sugar control is far more profound than most realise. Poor sleep doesn't just leave you tired, it fundamentally alters how your body processes glucose. When you don't get enough quality sleep, your cells become temporarily insulin resistant, making it harder for your body to manage blood sugar effectively.

Let's look at the science: Just one night of poor sleep can reduce insulin sensitivity by 25%; sleep deprivation increases stress hormones, which raise blood sugar; poor sleep affects hormones that control hunger and satiety; recovery from sleep debt can take multiple nights of good sleep.

This isn't just about feeling tired, it's about your body's fundamental ability to process energy. Think of good sleep as a reset button for your metabolism. Without it, your body's glucose management system operates like a computer running on low battery – everything slows down and becomes less efficient.

#PersonalTale

Through continuous glucose monitoring, I've watched this play out countless times. One poor night's sleep elevated my blood sugar levels for several days, even without changing diet or exercise. The data is striking; after a night of poor sleep, the same meal that usually causes minimal impact can trigger significant spikes.

The Breakfast Revelation.

Your first meal sets your metabolic tone for the day. A high-protein, low-sugar breakfast can improve your blood sugar control for the entire day. Skip the sugary cereals and reach for eggs, avocado or Greek yoghurt instead, with nuts and seeds.

Monitor to Motivate.

Everyone responds differently to foods. What spikes one person's blood sugar might not affect another's. This is why personalised monitoring can be so valuable; it takes the guesswork out of eating.

Remember: Your weight isn't just about calories in and calories out. It's about hormonal balance, inflammation control and understanding your body's unique responses to food. Small, consistent changes in how you eat and move can have profound effects on your health, your weight and, yes, your skin's appearance, too.

Managing your blood sugar isn't about perfection, it's about progress and balance. Every small change helps reduce inflammation and supports not just your weight goals but your overall health and skin ageing, too.

#DrVixTakeaways

1. Obesity isn't just about weight, it creates a perfect storm of inflammation in your body. Excess fat cells act like tiny factories pumping out inflammatory chemicals (cytokines), which affect everything from how quickly your skin ages to how well it heals.

2. The numbers tell a sobering story: 64% of UK adults are now overweight or obese, with C-reactive protein (CRP) levels typically two to three times higher than those with a healthy BMI.

3. Blood sugar regulation is like a thermostat; when it's disrupted by constant high-glycaemic foods, it creates a cascade of problems. Insulin resistance doesn't just affect your weight, it triggers inflammatory pathways that can compromise collagen production, accelerating skin ageing.

4. Advanced glycation end-products (AGEs) are troublemakers in your skin. They're formed when glucose binds to proteins, creating damaged molecules that stiffen tissues and compromise collagen. The result? Accelerated ageing, decreased elasticity and slower wound healing.

5. And now for the good news! Small changes make a big difference. Timing your meals, walking after eating, eating protein before carbs and choosing low-GI foods can help manage blood sugar spikes. Remember: your skin keeps score of every sugar spike; each healthy choice counts toward both your weight and skin health goals.

CHAPTER 6:
THE GUT PLOT

Your Second Brain's Impact on Ageing

Have you ever had a 'gut feeling' about something? I get them all the time, a deep-down sense telling me not to treat particular patients as I won't ever meet their expectations or to buy that Gucci bag because, obviously, it's life changing. But here's the twist: those instincts might be more scientific than you think.

Your gut and brain are in constant conversation through what scientists call the gut-brain axis – a complex network of neural, hormonal and chemical signals. And your skin is part of this chat, too, forming what I like to call the body's most talkative trio. The next time you feel a 'gut instinct' bubbling up, remember it might just be the group chat between your gut, brain and skin, each with something to say!

When I explain this to patients in the clinic, I often start with this surprising and somewhat mind-blowing fact: your gut contains more neurons than your spinal cord. Yes, you read that right, your gut has its own 'brain'. Known as the enteric nervous system, this network of neurons operates semi-independently, communicating constantly with your actual brain through the vagus nerve. That 'gut feeling' you get isn't just metaphorical, it's a direct result of this gut-brain connection.

Your enteric nervous system runs through your digestive tract; it's a sophisticated control centre with over 100 million nerve cells, lining your gut from your oesophagus to your rectum. This network is constantly chatting with your brain, producing 90% of your serotonin – the so-called happiness hormone – and sending signals back to your brain about how you're doing.

So, if your gut's not happy, chances are, neither is your brain. This is why stress can trigger digestive issues, and digestive problems can make you feel anxious or down; it's a two-way conversation happening 24/7.

I see this play out constantly in real life. Take me, for example, before public speaking. Ten minutes prior, you'll find me in the ladies' room, my tummy in absolute knots. A classic example of this brain-gut chat in action!

This isn't just fascinating trivia to wow your friends at dinner parties with, it's the key to understanding the deeply intertwined relationship between your emotional state, stress levels and skin. Your gut, often called the 'second brain', doesn't just digest your food, it plays a starring role in regulating mood, immunity, and inflammation. And your skin? It's part of the conversation, too. Stress or poor gut health can lead to inflammation, which, in turn, can exacerbate conditions like acne, rosacea and premature ageing. It's a chain reaction: stress impacts the gut, the gut sends distress signals to the brain, and your skin bears the brunt of it all.

Understanding this gut-brain-skin axis is a game-changer. It shifts the focus from treating symptoms in isolation to addressing the whole system. By nurturing your gut – through diet, stress management and even probiotics – you're not just helping your digestion, you're improving your mood, calming inflammation and promoting healthier, more radiant skin.

The Gut Microbiome.
More trivia for you: your gut houses around 100 trillion micro-organisms collectively weighing about 2 kg – roughly the weight of a small melon. (I'm not sure I like this fact!) These bacteria aren't just passive residents, either, they're active contributors to your health, producing neurotransmitters, hormones and other signalling molecules that influence everything from your mood to your skin's collagen production.

The communication between your gut and skin is like an elaborate game of Chinese whispers, but instead of verbal messages, it uses chemical messengers called cytokines and neuropeptides.

Your gut microbiome isn't just about digestion, it's a sophisticated chemical factory that produces everything from vitamin K to serotonin. These microorganisms break down foods into metabolites that, when your gut microbiome is balanced, send out anti-inflammatory signals that help maintain your skin's health. But when things go wrong, it's Chinese whispers gone wrong – the messages get distorted, triggering inflammation and skin problems.

For example, certain gut bacteria process fibre into short-chain fatty acids like butyrate, which helps maintain your gut barrier function and has anti-inflammatory properties. When these good bacteria diminish – whether from antibiotics, stress or poor diet – it's like losing your skin's internal support system.

Imagine your body's inflammatory response as well-organised emergency services. When everything is functioning as it should, firefighters arrive promptly to put out a fire and leave as soon as the job is done. But when your gut microbiome is out of balance, they stay indefinitely, hosing down the area long after the flames are gone, and instead of protecting your body, they end up causing unnecessary damage to the surrounding structures, including your skin.

This isn't just theory. We can measure increased levels of inflammatory markers in the blood of patients with skin conditions like rosacea and acne. These same markers are also often elevated in people with gut imbalances, showing a clear connection between what's happening in your digestive system and what you see in the mirror.

This persistent inflammation starts in your gut but doesn't stay there. Your gut lining is a selective security barrier; when it becomes compromised (what we call 'leaky gut'), it's like having a broken security system that lets unwanted substances slip through. Inflammatory molecules then travel through your bloodstream, eventually showing up on your skin as redness, breakouts or accelerated ageing.

#PersonalTale

In clinic, I've seen remarkable improvements in skin conditions when we prioritise supporting beneficial bacteria, particularly for my patients with rosacea who are preparing for laser treatment. As part of their regimen, I recommend targeted probiotics to optimise outcomes.

Not all bacteria are created equal. Some strains deserve special recognition for their skin-supporting powers. *Lactobacillus* and *Bifidobacterium*, the superstars of the probiotic world, help maintain your gut barrier function and modulate immune responses. They're like skilled diplomats, helping maintain peace between your immune system and the environment.

For example, certain strains of *Lactobacillus* are known to help reduce inflammatory markers linked to atopic dermatitis, while *Bifidobacterium longum* assists in regulating sebum production – nature's own oil-control system, so great for acne patients. The scientific names might sound long and complicated, but their effects are simple and profound: healthier, calmer skin.

This approach reinforces how gut health and skin health are deeply intertwined, offering patients more holistic and lasting results.

The three-way communication system of the gut-brain-skin axis is more sophisticated than the world's most advanced computer network. Your gut sends signals to your brain through the vagus nerve (kind of a dedicated fibre-optic cable carrying millions of messages per second). These signals influence everything from stress responses to skin cell turnover. When you're stressed, it sends signals to alter your gut's bacterial composition, often favouring pro-inflammatory species. These changes can lead to increased intestinal permeability (that leaky gut we talked about), which then triggers skin inflammation. It's a vicious cycle: stress affects your gut, your gut affects your skin, and your skin's appearance can then increase your stress levels.

Now, here's where things get interesting – and perhaps a bit sci-fi. Scientists are exploring the possibility of microbiome transfers specifically for skin health. While we've seen success with faecal microbiota transplants for gut conditions (yes, that's exactly what it sounds like), skin microbiome transfers are the new frontier. (Personally, I don't think I would want someone else's poo transferred to my gut, but each to their own – it's out there!) The idea is to receive bacteria from someone with healthy skin to help with conditions like eczema and acne, like reseeding a patchy lawn with fresh grass – a bacterial beauty treatment backed by science instead of hype!

But don't rush to trade bacteria with your clear-skinned friends just yet. This is still experimental, and success requires creating the right environment for these beneficial strains to thrive.

#ActionableSteps

After years of seeing the gut-brain-skin connection in clinic, I've developed practical, results-driven approaches that go beyond the basics. Putting science into action, here's a systematic protocol to rebalance both gut and skin health:

Phase 1: The Reset.

First, we need to calm inflammation by giving your gut a chance to reset. This involves a short-term elimination of common trigger foods to give your gut a break. Think of it like rebooting your computer when things aren't working properly – sometimes you need to shut everything down before starting fresh.

The tricky part is that not all of these foods are inherently 'bad' – some are actually nutrient-rich and beneficial for many people. But, if you're sensitive to them, they can trigger an inflammatory response. It requires detective work, patience and systematic elimination. Typically, you remove suspected triggers for three to four weeks, then carefully reintroduce them one at a time while monitoring your skin's response. Keep a food diary during this process – your skin's reactions might surprise you!

#PersonalTale

In clinic, I've seen patients mystified by persistent inflammation despite eliminating obvious triggers. One memorable case involved a woman who ate tomatoes daily in her 'healthy' Mediterranean diet, not realising they were contributing to her skin issues.

While common triggers like dairy and gluten often make headlines, nightshade vegetables are frequently overlooked troublemakers. Nightshades are a family of plants that include: tomatoes, peppers (bell peppers, chili peppers, paprika), white potatoes (sweet potatoes are not nightshades), eggplants and goji berries. These contain compounds called alkaloids, which some people's bodies interpret as a threat, launching an inflammatory response that shows up on their skin.

Within weeks of eliminating nightshades, my client's complexion transformed.

Phase 2: Repair and Repopulate.

Once inflammation is reduced, it's time to repair the gut. There are key nutrients that act as building blocks, and while you can take supplements, I prefer getting it naturally through food:

Glutamine is like your gut's construction foreman, strengthening the walls and maintaining order. Homemade bone broth is your best bet – it's literally gut-healing liquid gold. If bone broth isn't your thing, you can build your glutamine reserves with grass-fed beef, wild-caught fish or even cottage cheese. For my vegetarian patients, I recommend loading up on dark leafy greens and legumes.

Making bone broth is simple but it's all about patience. Take quality bones (I prefer beef or free-range chicken), roast them until golden for extra flavour, then simmer low and slow with aromatics like onions, garlic and a splash of apple cider vinegar (which helps extract those precious minerals) for at least 24 hours – though I often let mine go for 48. The longer it simmers, the more collagen and nutrients you'll extract. The final product should be rich, gelatinous when cooled, and packed with skin-loving compounds.

#PersonalTale

My house doesn't exactly smell like a spa when I'm making my weekly batch, and my husband hates the smell, but my skin's glow makes up for it! I usually make a large amount on Sunday, to last the week. It's become quite the ritual in my kitchen.

Then there's zinc, your gut's repair specialist. Oysters are the superstar here; just six give you more zinc than you need in a day. Not an oyster fan? No problem. A handful of pumpkin seeds, some grass-fed beef or even a square of dark chocolate can help you hit your zinc goals. Yes, you heard right – chocolate can be medicinal!

Collagen is your body's scaffolding, supporting both gut and skin structure. While bone broth shows up again here (seriously, it's that good), you can also get collagen support from fish with edible bones – think sardines and anchovies. Even the skin and joints of your roast chicken are doing more good than you might think. For the veggies out there, mushroom broth, made with a mix of dried and fresh mushrooms (shiitake, porcini, cremini) is a good option.

Finally, let's talk about your gut's community – those beneficial bacteria that do everything from fighting inflammation to supporting your skin's glow. Different strains have different superpowers. *Lactobacillus rhamnosus* is like your skin's bodyguard, strengthening its barrier function; you'll find it in aged cheeses and traditional buttermilk. *Bifidobacterium longum* is your inflammation fighter, abundant in traditional miso and properly fermented sauerkraut. Meanwhile, *Lactobacillus plantarum* provides antioxidant support; look for it in traditional sourdough bread and naturally fermented olives. Fermented foods aren't just trendy, they're potent skin medicine when used correctly.

Timing also matters. Consuming kimchi or sauerkraut with protein-heavy meals helps break down the protein more efficiently, reducing the likelihood of inflammation-triggering, partially digested proteins entering your bloodstream. And here's the thing most people don't realise, these beneficial bacteria need their own food to thrive. That's where prebiotic foods come in. Think of them as fertiliser for your gut garden. Jerusalem artichokes, garlic, onions and green bananas all feed your beneficial bacteria, helping them flourish and work better.

The key here is choosing real, traditionally prepared foods. And look for unpasteurised versions when possible; they're the ones still containing all the beneficial bacteria your gut (and skin) will thank you for. Those mass-produced yoghurts with 'added probiotics' … they're not quite the same as naturally fermented foods that have been made the same way for generations.

Marketing would have you believe these sweet little bottles are miracle workers for your microbiome, but let's cut through the hype – they're more about clever advertising than actual benefits. Think about it, you're essentially drinking sugary milk with a few million bacteria. Sounds impressive, right?

Picture your gut as a bustling city with billions of microbial residents. Those probiotic drinks? They're like dropping a handful of tourists into Manhattan and expecting them to change the city's culture. Unfortunately, most of the bacteria don't survive your stomach acid, and the ones that do are often not the strains your gut really needs, and the sugar content can actually feed the problematic bacteria you're trying to control. It's like sending in reinforcements with supplies for the opposition!

Phase 3: Maintenance and Modulation.
Maintaining your gut's bacterial community doesn't have to be complex. I encourage patients to think seasonally about gut health, incorporating a variety of foods and practices throughout the year, much like our ancestors did.

The relationship between diet and skin health goes deeper than just 'eat healthy'. Each meal is an opportunity to influence your microbiome. And by understanding that certain foods act as natural pharmaceutical agents, capable of shifting your bacterial balance and, consequently, your skin's behaviour, you can set the foundation for lasting health and glowing skin.

Remember, supporting your gut health isn't about quick fixes, it's about creating an environment where beneficial bacteria want to set up home and stay awhile.

#ActionableSteps
After years of clinical experience, I've discovered that the most effective approach to supporting gut health starts with food and supplements.

Nature has already created the perfect delivery system for beneficial bacteria through traditionally fermented foods. I'm not talking about mass-produced versions with added vinegar or sugar; your gut needs the real deal:

- Traditional sauerkraut, naturally fermented with just salt and time.

- Authentic kimchi, traditionally fermented.

- Real kefir, unsweetened and alive with beneficial organisms.

- Natural yoghurt that's thick and tangy from proper fermentation.

These foods are powerful because they don't just contain probiotics, they also provide the perfect environment for these beneficial bacteria to thrive – complete ecosystems in a jar.

If you choose to supplement probiotics, strategy matters more than brand names. Here's what to look for:

- Soil-based organisms that can actually survive your stomach acid. They're the Navy SEALs of the probiotic world, built to survive and thrive in harsh conditions.

- Multiple strains to support diverse gut flora and a resilient community.

- High doses (in the billions, not millions).

Timing matters when it comes to probiotic supplements. Taking them away from meals/on an empty stomach gives these beneficial bacteria their best shot at establishing themselves in your gut's ecosystem, and be aware that your morning tea or coffee could be sabotaging their effectiveness. Probiotics are delicate living organisms; heat is their kryptonite. Wait at least 30 minutes either side of taking your probiotics to have any hot drinks.

Also, be sure to keep them stored in a cool place and keep an eye on the expiry date (dead probiotics are useless probiotics!).

#PersonalTale

I learned this the hard way; for months, I was taking my probiotics with my morning coffee, essentially neutralising their benefits. Once I started spacing them apart, I noticed a real difference in their effectiveness. Now I take mine mid-morning, when my coffee is a distant memory.

What truly makes a difference is nourishing the beneficial bacteria already present in your body. Think of it this way: rather than just introducing new bacteria, create a supportive environment where the good ones can naturally flourish. Focus on incorporating a variety of fibre-rich foods, resistant starch, colourful vegetables and polyphenol-packed options like berries and olive oil into your diet.

Interestingly, your morning coffee ritual is already supporting this ecosystem. Research from Professor Tim Spector and the ZOE team shows that coffee creates an environment where beneficial gut bacteria flourish, making your daily brew a simple but effective way to nurture your microbiome. And here's the surprising part: it doesn't matter whether you drink regular or decaf; both types nourish specific gut bacteria that thrive on coffee compounds, which then produce antioxidants that boost your immune system and metabolism (like rewarding the helpful residents of your gut's community).

Far from being a guilty pleasure, your daily cup actively supports both gut and skin health. Just remember: skip the sugar to maximise these benefits! And, for those who don't enjoy coffee, there are many other ways to support your gut health through diet and lifestyle choices.

Your microbiome is like a garden; it thrives with regular care, not occasional, drastic interventions. While those trendy probiotic drinks might feel like a quick fix, your gut and skin deserve a more holistic approach. Regular, small portions of fermented foods are more beneficial than occasional large servings; daily prebiotic fibre has a greater impact than sporadic mega-doses. And don't forget to make stress management a daily practice, not just a reaction to crisis moments.

Microbiome Skincare.

The most exciting developments in microbiome research centre around personalisation. We're moving beyond one-size-fits-all probiotics towards tailored solutions based on your individual bacterial fingerprint.

Imagine skincare that's customised to your skin's exact bacterial makeup. Scientists are developing technologies that can actually analyse your skin's microbiome in real time and recommend specific combinations for your unique needs. The next generation of skincare won't just include probiotics, it'll provide exactly the right nutrients to help your skin's beneficial bacteria thrive. Think of it as precision farming for your face.

Have you heard of postbiotics? These are the beneficial compounds that good bacteria produce. Rather than just adding the bacteria, scientists are learning to harness their helpful byproducts, like growing garden herbs' essential oils rather than the whole plant.

The most exciting aspect of this revolution isn't just about new products, it's about understanding skin health in a completely new way. We're learning that healthy skin isn't 'clean' skin, it's balanced skin; different areas of your face need different bacterial populations; your skin's microbiome changes with seasons, stress and even your menstrual cycle, and the right topical probiotics can help your skin adapt.

But creating effective probiotic skincare isn't simple; there will be multiple challenges ahead. These beneficial bacteria need to be stable enough to survive in the product, active when they reach your skin, able to work with your skin's natural processes and be combined with ingredients that don't compromise their effectiveness.

As we understand more about the skin's microbiome, skincare routines will become more sophisticated but potentially simpler. Instead of ten different products, you might use fewer that work more intelligently with your skin's natural processes.

The future of skincare isn't about covering up problems or stripping your skin bare – it's about creating an environment where your skin's natural health can flourish. Just as we've learned the importance of gut health for overall wellbeing, we're discovering that nurturing your skin's microbiome is key to achieving that healthy, radiant complexion we all desire.

DrVixTakeaways

1. Your gut is more than just a digestive system, it's your 'second brain' (with more neurons than your spinal cord), producing 90% of your serotonin and directly influencing your skin's health through the gut-brain-skin axis.

2. Your gut microbiome (weighing about 2 kg) is a sophisticated chemical factory. When it's balanced, it sends out anti-inflammatory signals that support skin health; when it's disrupted, it can trigger inflammation, leading to skin issues like acne, rosacea and premature ageing.

3. Don't waste money on sugary probiotic drinks. Instead, focus on real, traditionally fermented foods like natural sauerkraut, kimchi, real kefir and tangy yoghurt that provide both the beneficial bacteria and their preferred environment.

4. The key nutrients for gut-skin health are readily available in food: glutamine (bone broth, grass-fed meat), zinc (oysters, pumpkin seeds) and collagen (fish with edible bones, chicken skin). These act as your gut's construction and repair team.

5. Coffee lovers, rejoice! Your morning brew (even decaf) creates a thriving environment for beneficial bacteria, supporting both gut and skin health – just skip the sugary additions that could counteract the benefits.

CHAPTER 7:
FOOD FOR THOUGHT, WRINKLES FOR FREE

What You Put on Your Plate Affects Your Skin

Your grandparents would likely be baffled by half the items in your shopping trolley today – and your body probably feels just as confused. In the span of just 150 years, humanity has dramatically transformed its eating habits. Modern manufacturing has fundamentally altered our relationship with food; while we've gained convenience, we've sacrificed the natural balance that sustained human health for centuries.

Ultra-processed foods (UPFs) have been modified so extensively that our bodies barely recognise them as food anymore. These products typically share concerning characteristics: they're high in omega-6 fatty acids from industrial seed oils, loaded with advanced glycation end-products (AGEs), stripped of natural nutrients and engineered to bypass our satiety signals (making it all too easy to keep eating without feeling full). Second helpings, anyone? The result is that only about 30% of people now eat two proper meals a day, with the rest relying on nutritionally deficient snacks to make up a quarter of their daily calories.

So, why are our supermarket shelves filled with UPFs? The uncomfortable truth is that they're cheap to produce and even cheaper to store. Manufacturers can take low-cost ingredients like refined flour, industrial seed oils and sugar, and turn them into products with almost endless shelf lives and impressive profit margins.

A ready-meal might cost you £2, while the fresh ingredients to cook it from scratch might cost triple that. That £2 ready-meal might look like a bargain, but it's a 'Buy Now, Pay Later' scheme – the real cost isn't on the price tag. You've seen it everywhere from all-inclusive hotel buffets to school canteens – the world of beige food. These pale, processed offerings might fill stomachs, but they're nutritionally bankrupt, promoting inflammation and disrupting our gut microbiome. When I see a beige buffet, I see a missed opportunity for vibrant, nutrient-rich foods that could actually support our health rather than compromise it.

Think of UPFs as taking out a high-interest loan on your health. Absolutely, that ready-meal saves you money and time today, but your body will be paying the inflammatory 'interest' for years to come. And trust me, this loan shark doesn't just want a little extra, it comes with an inflammatory interest rate that would make even my mortgage broker blush: increased inflammation, accelerated ageing and compromised health.

The terms 'processed' and 'ultra-processed' are often seen in a negative light, but what do they really mean? Are all processed foods actually bad for you?

Unless you're eating freshly harvested broccoli straight from your garden, most of the food you consume undergoes some level of processing – and that's not inherently a bad thing. Processing refers to altering a food's natural state to improve its shelf life, safety, taste or even its nutritional value. Methods like pasteurising, fermenting, freezing, canning and drying are all common forms of processing.

When it comes to ultra-processed foods, however, things take a turn. UPFs involve industrial techniques and ingredients that you wouldn't find in a typical home kitchen, which significantly diminish nutritional value while adding unhealthy components.

The NOVA Food Classification System categorises food into four groups based on how much processing they've undergone:

1. **Unprocessed or Minimally Processed Foods:** These are as close to their natural state as possible. Examples include washed and bagged spinach, pre-cut fresh fruit and frozen

vegetables. They are processed for convenience but retain their original nutritional value.

2. **Processed Culinary Ingredients:** These are derived from unprocessed foods using basic methods. Oils, butter, sugar, salt, dried herbs and spices fall into this group. They're not consumed on their own but are used to prepare other foods.

3. **Processed Foods:** These are made by combining minimally processed ingredients with sugar, oil, fat or salt. Examples include cheese, artisanal bread and tofu. These foods may be altered, but they are generally still nutritious and not harmful.

4. **Ultra-Processed Foods:** UPFs go through extensive industrial processes such as hydrogenation or moulding and include additives like stabilisers, emulsifiers, dyes and flavour enhancers. Examples include cookies, chips, fast food and sodas. These foods are often calorie-dense with little to no nutritional value and are engineered for convenience, taste and profitability.

The longer shelf life means these foods can sit in warehouses and on shelves for months, or even years. Natural food spoils – it's supposed to. When something can outlast your kitchen renovations, it's worth asking why.

While some processing is beneficial and necessary, UPFs can negatively impact your health when consumed in excess. They're designed to be hyper-palatable and convenient, but their nutritional drawbacks make it essential to limit them in your diet.

Group 1	Group 2	Group 3	Group 4
Unprocessed or Minimally Processed foods	Processed Culinary Ingredients	Processed Foods	Ultra-Processed Foods
fresh, dry, frozen vegetables or fruit, grains, legumes, meat, fish, eggs, nuts and seeds	Plant oils (eg. olive oil, coconut oil) animal fats (eg. cream, butter, lard, maple syrup, sugar, honey, and salt)	Canned/pickled vegetables, meat, fish, or fruit, artisanal bread, cheese, salted meats, wine, beer, and cider	Sugar sweetened beverages, sweet and savory packaged snacks, reconstituted meat products, pre-prepared frozen dishes, canned/instant soups, chicken nuggets, ice cream.
Processing includes removal of inedible/unwanted parts. Does not add substances to the original food.	Substances derived from Group 1 foods or from nature by processes including pressing, refining, grinding, milling, and drying.	Processing of foods from Group 1 or 2 with the addition of oil, salt, or sugar by means of canning, pickling, smoking, curing, or fermentation.	formulations made from a series of processes including extraction and chemical modification, includes very little intact Group 1 foods

Increasing Level of Processing →

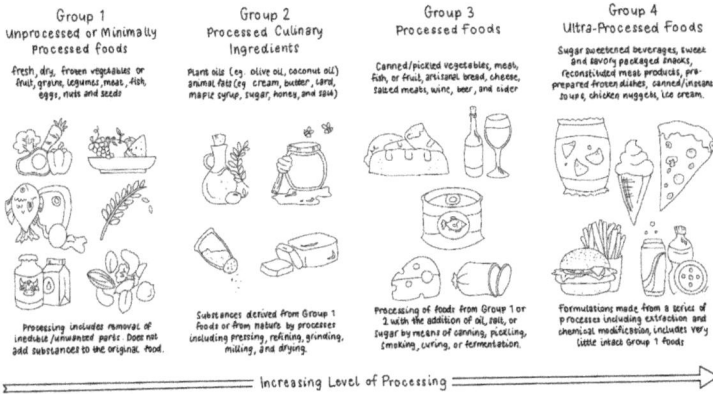

The Nova Guide to Processed Food

The UPF Reality: More Science Than Cooking.

What is really happening in those food factories?

UPFs aren't just ready-meals and fizzy drinks, they're the result of industrial processes that would look more at home in a chemistry lab than your kitchen. Imagine walking down your local supermarket's cereal aisle. They're not just grains anymore; they've been stripped, modified, bleached, fortified and sprayed with synthetic vitamins before being shaped into those appealing little Os and flakes. That 'wholegrain' claim on the box? It's a bit like putting a plaster on a broken arm – technically present, but not quite doing the job nature intended.

Let me give you an example. Picture a standard loaf of pre-packed, sliced, white bread – not the fresh, crusty kind from your local artisan bakery, but the kind that somehow stays soft and devoid of mould for weeks. Real bread goes stale and mouldy (trust me, my bread bin is practically a petri dish for penicillin every week). But this stuff? It's loaded with dough conditioners, preservatives and emulsifiers for that almost supernatural shelf life. And guess what? Your body gets to tackle all these strange, lab-made ingredients that our ancestors never encountered before you've even had your morning coffee.

Like fake-healthy cereals, another pet hate of mine are those 'healthy' protein bars millennials can't get enough of. Please, just take a look at the ingredients: modified starches, isolated proteins, artificial sweeteners, more sugars and a cocktail of gums and stabilisers. Yes, they're fortified with vitamins and minerals, but that's a bit like spray-painting nutrients on to barren soil; it's just not the same as getting them from real wholefoods.

With all this in mind, the real problem isn't just what's been added, it's what's been taken away. UPFs have been stripped of their bitter compounds (which often have health benefits), natural fibre (which feeds your gut bacteria) and the food matrix (how nutrients naturally occur together), then rebuilt like food Frankenstein's monsters.

Another problem – they're designed to be yummy. That perfect crunch of a crisp, the way certain snacks seem to dissolve on your tongue, the exact balance of sweet and salt in your favourite popcorn – none of this is accidental. Food scientists spend years perfecting these characteristics to override your body's natural satiety signals. And the truly insidious part? They're designed to be addictive. The perfect combination of salt, sugar and fat has been calculated to hit your pleasure centres like a flavour nuclear bomb. Your body's natural 'I'm full' signals don't stand a chance – well, this is my husband's excuse when he devours a whole packet of chocolate digestives.

The solution isn't about perfection, it's about awareness and making better choices.

Start reading labels. If you can't pronounce most of the ingredients, or if the list is longer than a Shakespearean sonnet, it's probably ultra-processed. Look for foods with ingredients you could buy yourself, or, better yet, choose foods that don't need ingredient lists – honestly, when was the last time you saw a nutrition label on a carrot?

Remember: Every time you shop, you're voting with your wallet for the kind of food system you want. The more we understand UPFs, the better equipped we are to make choices that support our health rather than food industry profits.

Advanced Glycation End-Products (AGEs).

Did you know that, beyond exposure to UPFs, there are also 'hidden agers' lurking in your food? Yes, it gets worse.

(Despite knowing this, what did I choose for breakfast this morning? Delicious, crispy bacon. Bacon actually scores a big fat zero on my ZOE app as do all my yummy charcuterie board favourites.)

AGEs (the 'hidden agers') can form inside our bodies as well as exist in certain foods, especially those that are highly processed or heavily cooked. They are basically like unwanted glue in your system that form when sugar molecules, floating around in your bloodstream (especially when blood sugar is high), stick to proteins or fats. It's like having tiny pieces of tape randomly attaching themselves to important structures in your body, making them stiff and less functional.

Your body perceives AGEs as unwelcome invaders, sparking an inflammatory response. Think of it as having countless microscopic splinters lodged in your system – your body is in a constant battle to remove them, resulting in ongoing inflammation. This chronic inflammatory state not only accelerates ageing but also plays a role in the development of various diseases.

In short, AGEs are unwanted souvenirs of cooking that are secretly ageing us. You know that delicious browning that happens when you toast bread, the irresistible crunch of crispy bacon, those perfectly golden roast potatoes, a smoky, charred BBQ steak or creamy caramelised onions (yes, all the foods that make life worth living!) … That's not just cooking, it's glycation, happening right before your eyes and creating AGEs. And every time you enjoy these foods, you're essentially inviting more of these ageing accelerators to take up residence in your tissues.

The real trouble comes when dietary AGEs collide with the ones your body creates due to high blood sugar. This double hit is a major accelerator of ageing, like pressing fast-forward on your body's ageing process. When you eat foods high in AGEs while your blood sugar is elevated, you're not just adding to your AGE burden, you're multiplying it.

#PersonalTale

I learned this the hard way during my continuous glucose monitoring experiment. My weekend indulgence of crispy bacon and toast didn't just taste good, it created a perfect AGE storm in my body. My skin actually looked different the next day.

And now I know why: I had unknowingly maxed out my AGE production, both from my food choices and my blood sugar response.

By the way, I apologise if this chapter feels a bit bleak, but try and consider it a wake-up call, an opportunity to gain insights that could truly make a difference!

Now you can see why my ZOE app gives bacon a zero rating – it's not just about the fat or salt content, but also about these ageing compounds that form during the cooking process.

And, I'm sorry, but AGEs aren't working alone. Their partners in crime, advanced lipoxidation end-products (ALEs), form when fats oxidise. These compounds form when oils are heated repeatedly – chip shop oil is the worst offender because it's been used over and over again. ALEs create chain reactions of damage in your cells and are abundant in processed foods. What's worse, they can form even during storage, meaning that bottle of vegetable oil in your cupboard might be accumulating ALEs as it sits there.

But don't worry, all this doesn't mean you need to eat everything boiled and bland. Understanding AGEs and ALEs is about making informed choices and finding clever ways to enjoy your favourite foods while minimising their impact. Because, let's be honest, life's too short for completely boring food, but it's also too precious to unknowingly accelerate ageing.

#ActionableSteps

So, how can you outsmart these ageing villains?

Start by cutting down on high-sugar and high-carb foods like pastries, sugary drinks and white bread. Instead, replace them with nutrient-dense options that nourish your skin from the inside out. Fruits and vegetables are your skin's artillery; packed with antioxidants, vitamins and minerals, they fight free radicals, offering a protective shield against premature ageing.

- **Berries:** Blueberries, strawberries and raspberries are antioxidant powerhouses, rich in vitamins C and E, which help to repair and rejuvenate your skin.

- **Leafy Greens:** Spinach, kale and Swiss chard are loaded with vitamins A and C, crucial for collagen production and skin repair.

- **Citrus Fruits:** Oranges, lemons and grapefruits are high in vitamin C, which not only boosts collagen synthesis but also brightens your complexion.

- **Nuts and seeds:** Almonds, chia seeds and flaxseeds are great sources of essential fatty acids, which help maintain skin elasticity and hydration.

A well-balanced diet is key. Aim for a plate that is vibrant and varied:

- **Half Plate:** Fill half of your plate with a colourful array of fruits and vegetables.

- **Quarter Plate:** Add a serving of lean protein like chicken, tofu and beans, which provide the building blocks for collagen and repair.

- **Quarter Plate:** Choose wholegrains or complex carbs such as quinoa, brown rice and sweet potatoes, which offer sustained energy and help manage blood sugar levels.

- **Don't forget hydration!** Drinking plenty of water helps to keep your skin plump and flushes out toxins. You can also hydrate your skin with water-rich fruits like cucumbers and melons.

HEALTHY PLATE RULE

VEGETABLES & FRUITS

Vegetables and fruits – ½ of your plate. Aim for colour & variety, eat the rainbow & remember that potatoes don't count as vegetables on the Healthy Eating Plate because of their negative impact on blood sugar.

PROTEIN SOURCES

Fish, poultry, beans, and nuts are all healthy, versatile protein sources—they can be mixed into salads, and pair well with vegetables on a plate. Limit red meat, and avoid processed meats such as bacon and sausage.

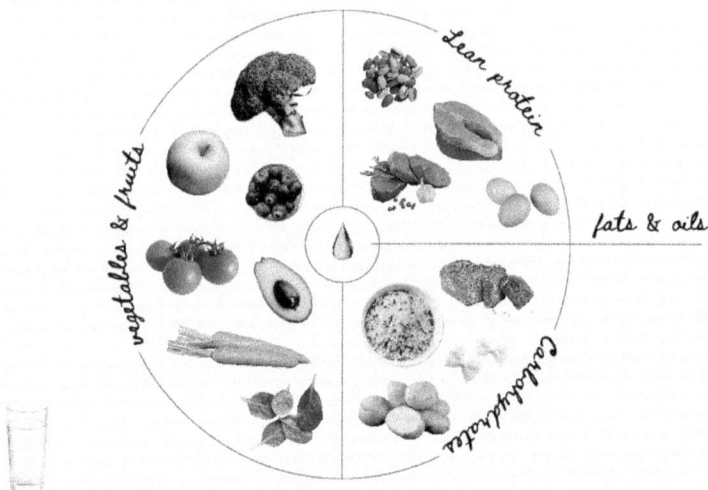

LIQUIDS

Skip sugary drinks, limit milk and dairy products to one to two servings per day, and limit juice to a small glass per day.

FATS & OILS

Nuts, avocados and olive oils.

CARBOHYDRATES

Go for whole grains – ¼ of your plate. — whole wheat, barley, quinoa, oats, brown rice, and foods made with them, such as whole wheat pasta—have a milder effect on blood sugar and insulin than white bread, white rice,

Dr Vix Manning

Your Healthy Plate

Remember: what you put on your plate is just as important as what you put on your skin. Incorporating these dietary changes consistently can transform your skin from tired and dull to radiant and youthful. By focusing on a diet rich in antioxidants and low in sugar, you're giving your skin the tools it needs to stay vibrant and fresh for years to come.

So, the next time you reach for that sugary treat, consider the long-term effects on your skin and opt for a healthier alternative instead. Your future self will thank you!

After decades in clinical practice and experiencing my own nutritional wake-up calls, here are some practical tips:

- Cook from scratch when you can and use raw ingredients.

- Read labels like a detective.

- Choose foods that rot.

- Make friends with your local greengrocer.

Your body is still running on ancient software in a modern nutritional world. While we can't change evolution, we can make choices that help our bodies thrive despite these challenges.

#DrVixTakeaways

1. Your shopping trolley is your crystal ball – what you put in it today predicts your health tomorrow. While that ultra-processed microwave meal might be cheap and convenient now, it's like taking out a high-interest loan against your future health.

2. Modern food manufacturing has transformed our relationship with food. Our bodies are confused by UPFs that are engineered to be addictive, bypass our satiety signals and stay 'fresh' for unnaturally long periods. If it doesn't spoil in your pantry, ask yourself why.

3. Those deliciously crispy, browned foods (like my breakfast bacon!) are loaded with AGEs. When combined with high blood sugar, they create a perfect storm of ageing compounds in your body.

4. Your plate should be your palette: half colourful fruits and vegetables (nature's anti-ageing arsenal), a quarter lean protein (your collagen building blocks) and a quarter complex carbs (for sustained energy). Think rainbow, not beige!

5. You don't need to be perfect – progress beats perfection. Small, consistent changes yield significant results.

PART THREE:

The Environmental Ageing Matrix

CHAPTER 8:
THE OMEGA EFFECT

Balancing Your Body's Inflammation Scales

I'm genuinely excited to share this chapter with you because balancing omega fats has genuinely transformed my family's quality of life – from significantly improving our sleep patterns to dramatically reducing niggling aches and pains we'd all come to accept as 'normal'. What started as a clinical exploration became a personal revelation that changed how I approach both my patients' health and my own family's wellbeing.

The modern food landscape is a paradox. While our supermarkets are bursting with more choices than ever, finding truly nourishing food has become surprisingly challenging. Our shelves are stocked with products that are masterpieces of convenience but nutritional deserts – high in sugar, low in fibre and engineered for taste rather than health.

But here's the exciting part: we're also living in an era of unprecedented nutritional knowledge. Science has given us the ability to understand our unique nutritional needs with remarkable precision. No more guesswork, no more generic advice and definitely no more random buying of supplements based on the latest social media trend. Today, we can create personalised plans that are like having a precision GPS for nutrition. The best part? This targeted approach often means fewer supplements, better results and no more expensive trial and error.

Intrigued? Well, read on, we are now going to talk about fats, but not in the way you might expect. I want you to forget everything you've heard about 'good fats' and 'bad fats' for a moment, because I'm going to share something that transformed how I think about fats entirely. You see, it's not just about choosing the right fats, it's about getting them in the right balance. And trust me, this balance is probably more off-kilter than you imagine.

When I first tested my own omega ratios, I was genuinely shocked. Despite eating what I considered a healthy diet (yes, even with the occasional chocolate biscuit), taking regular fish oil supplements, and generally making good choices, my omega-6 to omega-3 ratio was a whopping 17:1. That's not just slightly out of balance, that's a full-blown inflammatory disaster! And I'm not alone – 97% of the population show similar patterns, regardless of how 'clean' they believe their diets to be.

This discovery was both humbling and liberating. Humbling because it showed me that even as a doctor, I'd been missing something fundamental about nutrition. Liberating because it gave me a clear, measurable target to adjust. Within three months of strategic omega balancing, those mysterious joint pains that had plagued me simply vanished. And my husband's sleep quality improved dramatically – he was finally getting that deep, restorative sleep he'd been missing.

What makes the omega story so compelling isn't just the science (though it's fascinating, and we'll get to it), it's how quickly and noticeably it can transform how you feel. When you correct severe omega imbalances, the effects can be profound and surprisingly swift. It's one of the few nutritional interventions where patients often report 'feeling different' within weeks.

So, let's dive into the omega effect – a nutritional approach that might just be the missing piece in your inflammation puzzle. I promise to keep it practical, actionable and free from unnecessary complexity. Because ultimately, this isn't about sticking to complicated plans, it's about making informed tweaks that can dramatically shift your inflammatory balance and, quite possibly, how you feel every single day.

Your body's fat balance is like a well-tuned system. When everything is aligned, your skin radiates, inflammation stays in check and your cells perform at their best. However, in today's modern world, this natural balance has been severely thrown off.

Going back a few years: Our ancestors evolved on a diet with a near-equal balance of essential fats. They didn't plan it that way, it was simply the natural ratio found in wild game, fish and foraged foods. Fast forward to today, and our food supply has undergone a radical transformation. The introduction of industrial seed oils, factory farming, processed foods and even some so-called health foods has disrupted the equilibrium that kept us thriving for centuries, sending our omega-6 levels soaring while our omega-3 intake has plummeted.

Consider your omega-6 to omega-3 ratio as a vital health metric, like blood pressure or cholesterol levels. When balanced, it promotes wellness and reduces inflammation; when out of balance, it invites inflammation, ageing and chronic illness.

As I mentioned, despite years of faithfully taking fish oil and eating what I thought was a healthy diet, my ratio was still 17:1, which is awful but unfortunately an average figure these days. This discovery pushed me to dig deeper into omega science and ultimately helped me understand why conventional supplementation often falls short.

The ghastly fish oil capsules you swallow every morning are a small floodgate against a massive wave of omega-6 that floods in from our food supply. For it to work effectively, we must seal the leaks by reducing omega-6 intake, choosing quality omega-3s and verifying progress through testing.

In today's world, balancing your omegas isn't just a choice, it's a modern necessity for reducing inflammation, promoting healthy ageing and protecting your overall health.

#ActionableSteps

At the end of the book, I'll give you a QR code where I can recommend a safe and affordable way to test your levels.

Why does this matter to you? This imbalance isn't just a nutritional number, it's a key driver of chronic inflammation. Did you know that for optimal cellular health and minimal inflammation, your ratio should be 3:1, but the shocking reality is most people are running closer to 25:1!

Think about that for a moment. Even if you are doing 'everything right' – eating fish regularly and taking fish oil supplements – you will often find yourself far from this optimal ratio. And it's not your fault; our modern food system, with its abundance of 'yummy' processed foods and industrial seed oils, has tilted this balance dramatically.

Why does this matter for ageing? When your omega ratio is out of balance, your cells essentially marinate in inflammatory signals. This affects everything from your skin's collagen production to your brain function. Getting this ratio closer to the ideal 3:1 starts with controlling one of ageing's major accelerators.

We know your skin reflects what's happening inside your body. When there's too much omega-6, your skin becomes more prone to inflammation, which can accelerate ageing and worsen conditions like acne, eczema and rosacea.

Finally, your heart and blood vessels rely on a healthy omega balance too. An excess of omega-6 can increase inflammation in your blood vessels, making them stiffer and increasing the risk of heart disease. So, you are adding extra stress to your circulatory system, which can lead to serious health issues.

In essence, when omega-6 dominates, your body feels the effects across multiple areas, from cellular health to your brain, skin and heart. The right balance helps keep these systems running smoothly and lowers inflammation, promoting overall wellness.

DHA (Docosahexaenoic Acid).
Imagine your cell membranes as bustling construction sites. Essential fatty acids, like omega-6 and omega-3, serve as the raw materials for building these structures, but they each create very different 'buildings'. Omega-6, for instance, is pro-inflammatory, while omega-3 is anti-inflammatory. Think of them as teammates that ideally work together, but when one side is overrepresented, things start to go wrong; when omega-6 takes over, you have too many demolition crews and not enough builders – it disrupts balance and promotes inflammation.

Let me walk you through what happens in your body when there's an imbalance between omega-6 and omega-3 fatty acids:

First, your cell membrane flexibility changes. Your cell membranes are like thin, flexible walls that need to stay soft and permeable. When you have an excess of omega-6, these walls become more rigid and less flexible. This makes it harder for cells to let nutrients in, send signals (like hormones) and flush out toxins. In short, your cells struggle to function efficiently.

Next is your brain health. Your brain is a major fan of omega-3, especially a type called DHA (docosahexaenoic acid), and for good reason. DHA makes up about 30% of your brain's grey matter; it literally helps build the structure of your brain! Think of DHA as your brain's favourite building material. Just as you'd want the highest quality materials when building a house, your brain specifically seeks out DHA to construct and maintain its cells. When you're running low on DHA, it's like trying to renovate a house with substandard materials; things just don't work as well as they should. If there's too much omega-6, your cognitive function can suffer.

So, what makes DHA so special for your brain?

It helps your brain cells communicate effectively – akin to having a perfect Wi-Fi signal instead of that frustrating buffering. It supports the formation of new neural connections –new roads and pathways in your brain. It helps protect your existing brain cells from damage – a high-tech security system for your neurons. It's crucial for memory formation and recall – your brain's filing system works better with adequate DHA.

When your omega-6 levels are too high, they literally compete with DHA for space in your brain cells. Even if you're taking DHA supplements or eating fatty fish, if your omega-6 levels are through the roof, it's harder for that precious DHA to get where it needs to go.

I see this all the time, patients complaining about brain fog, poor concentration or memory issues not realising that their omega imbalance might be contributing to these problems. In fact, one serving of chips fried in vegetable oil can deliver more omega-6 than our ancestors consumed in an entire week! Scary fact!

The good news? Once you understand this balance, you can take strategic steps to improve it, and your brain is remarkably responsive to improvements in DHA levels. Remember, this isn't about quick fixes, but making informed choices that support your body's natural anti-inflammatory processes.

#ActionableSteps

One of the best food sources of omega-3 is wild-caught fatty fish (salmon, mackerel, sardines). It is important, though, to understand the difference between wild-caught and farmed salmon, because it's not just about taste – it's about fundamental nutrition. When a salmon swims freely in the ocean, it feeds on a diet of smaller fish, krill and algae – all rich in omega-3s – creating flesh packed with these beneficial fats in their most natural form. On the flip side, farmed salmon are typically fed processed pellets often made from corn and soy, and can have up to 50% less omega-3 content than their wild counterparts. Even more concerning, they tend to be higher in pro-inflammatory omega-6s from their grain-based diet. Think about it, we're essentially feeding farmed fish the same inflammatory diet that's causing problems in us!

While farmed salmon is certainly better than no salmon, if you're trying to optimise your omega-3 levels, wild-caught makes a significant difference. If you can't get wild salmon? Consider smaller fish like sardines and mackerel, which are usually wild-caught and have the added benefit of being lower in environmental toxins.

Interestingly, all fish get their omega-3s from algae – they're the middlemen in this nutritional chain. That's why algae supplements can be a fantastic option, especially for vegetarians, vegans and those concerned about fish sustainability.

Also good are fish eggs (caviar, if you're feeling fancy!) and high-quality fish oil supplements (look for ones with a high DHA content).

Remember though, it's not just about adding more DHA, it's about creating the right environment for it to work effectively. This means reducing competing omega-6s and ensuring your overall fatty acid balance is optimal. You need to clear the traffic so that DHA can reach its destination – your brain cells – more easily.

EPA (Eicosapentaenoic Acid).

So, we have discussed DHA, now let's look at EPA, the unsung hero of the omega-3 family. While DHA tends to steal the spotlight with its brain-boosting benefits, EPA quietly works behind the scenes as your body's anti-inflammation conductor, orchestrating a complex symphony of responses.

Think back to the last time you had a flare-up, whether it was angry skin, aching joints or muscles or even a low mood. EPA acts like your body's natural firefighter, rushing to calm these inflammatory hot spots. And what makes it particularly remarkable is its versatility; not only does it compete with those troublesome omega-6s but it also helps produce specialised compounds called resolvins that actively cool inflammation.

Even more than that, EPA doesn't just fight the inflammation, it helps prevent it from flaring up in the first place. It's like having a skilled diplomat in your body, maintaining peace before conflicts arise. This is why maintaining optimal EPA levels is so important and creates a more resilient system overall.

Another fact: simply popping an omega-3 supplement often isn't enough to fix this imbalance. Unfortunately, most supplements are underdosed. Many fish oil supplements don't provide sufficient DHA and EPA, the active forms of omega-3 your body needs. You might think you're getting enough, but the dose may be far too low.

Supplementation.

The fish oil capsule you may be taking might say '1000 mg' on the label, but here's the reality check: only a portion of that is actual EPA and DHA. Typical 1000 mg fish oil capsules might contain only 180 mg EPA and around 120 mg DHA. As for the rest? It's other fats and filler oils.

Research suggests that for anti-inflammatory benefits, you might need 1000–2000 mg of EPA and 500–1000 mg of DHA daily. Do the maths; that single capsule isn't cutting it. You'd need to take a handful to reach therapeutic doses. No wonder so many people say fish oil 'doesn't work' for them!

Remember, quality *and* quantity matter here. A high-quality supplement at the right dose can make a remarkable difference to your inflammatory balance, skin health and overall wellbeing.

So, not all omega-3s are created equal when it comes to absorption and effectiveness. The form in which they are delivered makes a big difference to how well your body can use them. For example, omega-3s in their natural triglyceride form are closer to how they're found in whole foods, like fish, which makes them easier for your body to recognise and absorb. In contrast, many cheaper omega-3 supplements come in an ethyl ester form, which requires extra processing by the body before it can be absorbed. This difference may not sound like much, but it can impact how much omega-3 actually gets into your cells.

The best omega-3 also comes bound to compounds like polyphenols (naturally occurring plant compounds with anti-oxidant properties). Omega-3s in whole foods, like salmon and anchovies, are often found with polyphenols and other nutrients that protect omega-3s from breaking down too quickly and make them more bioavailable – meaning your cells can absorb and use them more effectively. In essence, you get a higher-quality dose directly to where it's needed most, with the added bonus of reduced oxidation (which can make omega-3s less effective over time).

However, remember that even high-quality omega-3 can't compete if you're consistently eating excessive omega-6 in your diet. Modern diets are a minefield of hidden omega-6 sources, making it nearly impossible to maintain an ideal ratio without intentional changes.

Let's look at some major culprits:

Vegetable oils. Soybean, corn, sunflower, safflower and cottonseed oils are standard in many snacks, sauces and convenience meals. These might help extend shelf-life and enhance texture, but they also flood our diets with omega-6, tipping the balance and increasing the risk of chronic inflammation. Most restaurants use industrial seed oils for cooking, so even seemingly healthy dishes can come drenched in omega-6s, setting back your balance.

Nuts and seeds, while beneficial in moderation, are also naturally high in omega-6. Overconsumption of these, too, can disrupt the optimal ratio.

Achieving an omega balance requires a strategic approach focused on both reducing omega-6 and increasing omega-3. But here's the key: it needs to be systematic, monitored and tailored to ensure it's effective.

#ActionableSteps

Start by identifying and cutting back on omega-6-heavy foods. Switch out vegetable oils for olive or avocado oil, and be mindful of omega-6-rich snacks.

Then, boost your omega-3 intake. Look for high-quality omega-3 supplements that offer sufficient DHA and EPA in a highly absorbable form. Focus on eating more fatty fish like wild salmon, mackerel and sardines as well.

And finally, test, don't guess. Without testing, you're working in the dark. Regular omega ratio testing allows for targeted interventions, ensuring that your efforts to balance omegas are effective. Scan the QR code at the end of the book to learn about our clinically validated testing options that help optimise your supplementation strategy.

So, here's the bottom line – and I say this not just as a doctor, but as someone who's been on this journey myself – achieving the right omega balance in today's world isn't just about adding more fish oil to your diet, it's about understanding the bigger picture and making strategic changes that actually work.

Remember, this isn't about perfection, it's about progress. Your body is constantly working to maintain balance but it needs a little help. Give it the right tools and it will reward you with better health, slower ageing and, yes, even better skin.

#DrVixTakeaways

1. Your omega balance isn't just a number, it's a crucial health metric as important as your blood pressure or cholesterol. Modern diets send our omega-6 to omega-3 ratio soaring to 15:1 or higher, when historically it was closer to 1:1. This is a major driver of inflammation and ageing.

2. The fish oil capsule you're taking, it's probably not enough. Most supplements are seriously underdosed; you need to look for the actual EPA and DHA content, not just the total oil amount. Think of it like trying to fill a swimming pool with a teaspoon – the material is right, but the dose is way off.

3. DHA is your brain's favourite building material, making up 30% of your brain's grey matter. But here's the catch: when omega-6 levels are too high, they compete with DHA for space in your brain cells, affecting cognition.

4. Hidden omega-6 sources are everywhere from restaurant meals to those 'healthy' nuts and seeds – even farmed fish are high in omega-6 due to their grain-based feed. One serving of chips fried in vegetable oil can deliver more omega-6 than our ancestors consumed in a week!

5. Don't guess, test! Without measuring your omega ratio, you're working in the dark. Regular testing helps ensure your efforts to balance omegas are actually working, not just wishful thinking.

CHAPTER 9:
STRESS, SPIDERS
AND SPREADSHEETS

The Cortisol Connection

Have you ever looked in the mirror after a particularly chaotic week and thought, 'I've aged five years in five days'? Trust me, you're not imagining things – and it's not just the dark circles or the sudden breakout that appeared right before your important presentation.

What if I told you that the stress you're feeling is literally showing up on your face faster than any premium skin serum could possibly counteract? As both a doctor and someone who juggles way too many balls in the air at any one time – clinic hours, writing, family life and, yes, occasional Netflix binges (we all have our vices!) – I've seen firsthand how stress affects us.

The connection between stress and ageing isn't just anecdotal, it's biological. That fight-or-flight response that served our ancestors so well when escaping predators is now being triggered by your overflowing inbox, the school run and that passive-aggressive email from your colleague. The fascinating (and honestly, quite maddening) truth is that your body can't distinguish between running from a lion and running late for a meeting – it mobilises the same powerful hormonal cascade either way.

In this chapter, we're going to explore the remarkable science behind how stress hormones like cortisol are secretly sabotaging your skin's collagen, accelerating ageing and fuelling inflammation from the inside out. But don't worry, this isn't just a doom-and-gloom stress sermon. I'll share the strategies that have genuinely worked for my most stressed patients (and for me during those weeks when I'm burning the candle at both ends).

In our modern world, stress has become as familiar as the *ping* our phones make when we receive a message – an almost constant companion. While society has normalised living under pressure, our bodies haven't quite got the memo that not every deadline is a predator requiring a fight-or-flight response.

Unfortunately, the impact of this constant state of alert extends far deeper than the tension in your shoulders or that knot in your stomach. Behind every stressful meeting, your unread email list, or sleepless night, a complex cascade of hormones floods your system. Cortisol, adrenaline and noradrenaline – your body's stress response team – work overtime, causing changes that are meant to be temporary but have become chronic for many of us. This hormonal havoc doesn't just affect your mood or energy, it accelerates ageing at a cellular level, influences everything from your skin's repair mechanisms to your brain's cognitive function and can fundamentally alter how your body operates.

Understanding this intricate relationship between stress and your body's responses isn't just academic, it's essential for anyone seeking to maintain their health and slow the ageing process.

The Benefits of Stress.
Yes, stress can be beneficial; it activates our body's fight-or-flight response, helping us react quickly and effectively to challenges and dangers. It keeps us alive. Cortisol, adrenaline and noradrenaline are the key players.

When faced with stress, your adrenal glands (small organs sitting on top of your kidneys) release cortisol, often called the 'stress hormone'. This release happens through what's known as the hypothalamic-pituitary-adrenal (HPA) axis – a communication network between your brain and adrenal glands.

Once released into your bloodstream, cortisol triggers several metabolic changes:

1. It signals your liver to convert stored glycogen into glucose and release it into your bloodstream. It also reduces insulin

sensitivity in your tissues, which keeps blood glucose levels elevated.

2. This glucose surge provides immediate energy to your muscles, brain and other organs, preparing you to respond effectively to the stressful situation – whether that's fighting, fleeing or managing a challenging task.

3. Simultaneously, cortisol performs a dual role in your immune system: it provides the necessary energy (glucose) for immune cells to function properly during an inflammatory response, while also moderating that same inflammation to prevent it from becoming excessive. This dual action on inflammation is particularly important; cortisol acts as a short-term anti-inflammatory by suppressing certain immune functions and inflammatory pathways, which helps protect your body from the potential damage of an unchecked inflammatory response.

Adrenaline, in turn, speeds up your heart rate, directs blood flow to the muscles and relaxes your airways, enabling deeper breathing. This process improves oxygen supply to your muscles, preparing you to either run faster or confront a threat head-on. Noradrenaline complements this response by sharpening focus and heightening attention.

Together, these transmitters create a physiological state that equips you to respond effectively, whether by choosing to fight, flee or freeze when faced with a daunting challenge – like encountering Shelob (I'll explain this shortly).

The Negatives of Stress.
While cortisol can be beneficial in the short term, its effects can become detrimental over the longer term. Imagine living in a house where your burglar alarm never stops ringing. Chronic stress keeps your body's emergency systems blaring at full volume, day and night. While a brief burst of stress might help you escape that giant spider in your living room, constant stress is like having your body's ageing accelerator stuck on full throttle.

Stress can manifest in various ways, making it essential to recognise the symptoms to maintain your wellbeing.

Physically, you may experience headaches, muscle tension, aches and pains or abdominal pain – signals from your body that indicate the need for relaxation. Emotionally, stress can lead to anxiety, irritability, sadness and overwhelm, all of which can negatively impact your mood and daily functioning.

Brain function can also be affected. Your concentration may decrease, and routine tasks might feel overwhelming. Additionally, stress often disrupts sleep patterns. Normally, melatonin levels rise in the evening, signalling to our body that it's time to wind down. However, when cortisol levels are high due to stress, it can mess with melatonin production, making it harder to fall or stay asleep. This cycle of stress and sleep disruption is one that's tough to break.

Over time, chronic stress can have more serious consequences, potentially contributing to burnout, cardiovascular issues and a compromised immune system. It can really take a toll on our health, affecting everything from energy levels to emotional wellbeing.

Does any of this sound familiar? It's crucial to tackle stress head-on with a bit of self-care and some solid coping strategies because staying chill is the key to keeping healthy and resilient in the long run!

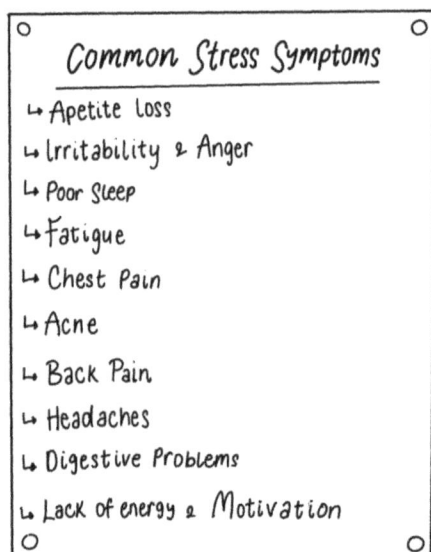

Common Stress Symptoms

↳ Apetite Loss

↳ Irritability & Anger

↳ Poor Sleep

↳ Fatigue

↳ Chest Pain

↳ Acne

↳ Back Pain

↳ Headaches

↳ Digestive Problems

↳ Lack of energy & Motivation

Common Stress Symptoms

#PersonalTale – The Doctor, the Spider and the Stress Response
So, onto the spider issue – my ultimate nemesis.

I have my mother to thank for this fear. As a child, about four years old, I'd be halfway up the stairs when, suddenly, she'd let out a blood-curdling shriek and pretend to be Shelob, the giant spider from *Lord of the Rings*.

Fast forward to adulthood, and there I am, peacefully watching *Vampire Diaries* on Netflix (my guilty pleasure), maybe with a cup of tea and a biscuit, when, out of the corner of my eye, I spot a spider the size of a small cow lurking ominously nearby. What happens next isn't just fear, it's my body flipping into full-on emergency mode, ready to face (or flee from) this eight-legged menace. In my case, the 'flight' part of 'fight or flight' wins every time. I'm out of that room faster than Usain Bolt in a sprint, leaving behind a trail of dust.

My mother's voice still echoes in my head: 'If you want to live and thrive, let a spider go alive.' But in that moment, my survival instinct cares little for ancient wisdom.

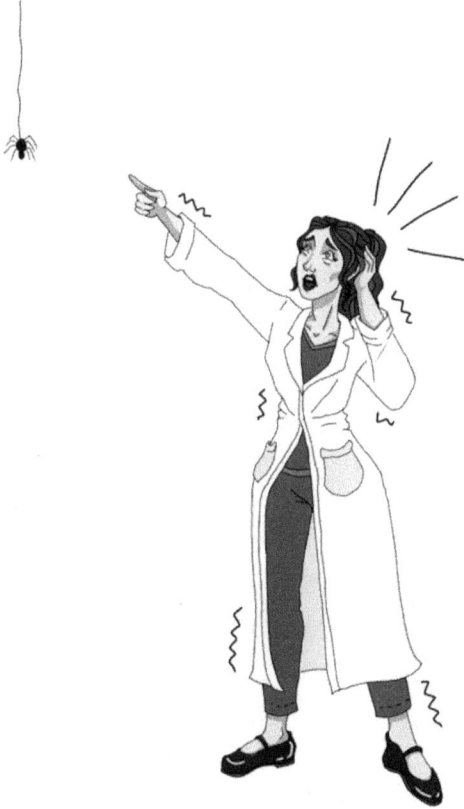

The Spider and Me

Joking aside, your body can't tell the difference between a massive arachnid and your mounting email inbox at work. To your internal alarm system, stress is stress. That looming work deadline? Your body treats it the same as being chased by a prehistoric predator. Upcoming mortgage payment? You might as well be facing a sabre-toothed tiger. And this is where things get problematic. While our stress response system was perfectly designed for our ancestors' immediate threats (run from predator, then relax), our modern stressors never seem to end: work stress flows into family responsibilities, which merge with financial worries, health concerns and that endless to-do list. Your body's alarm system never gets a chance to switch off. Does this sound all too familiar?

Stress in the Skin.

Consider your cells as millions of tiny batteries; each stressful event drains them a little. Usually, they recharge during periods of rest and recovery, but with chronic stress, they never return to full power. Instead, they start operating at a perpetual low-power mode, affecting everything from your skin's collagen production to your energy levels.

Remember those telomeres we talked about in Chapter 2? Stress takes scissors to these protective caps on your DNA, accelerating your cellular ageing clock.

Your skin is particularly chatty when it comes to revealing stress levels. That sudden breakout before an important presentation isn't a coincidence; cortisol triggers your oil glands to produce more sebum, essentially creating a perfect storm for acne. It also breaks down collagen, your skin's natural scaffolding. So, stress is basically playing a game of Jenga with your skin's support structure, gradually pulling away the pieces that keep everything firm and bouncy. Over time, this leads to more than temporary spots – we're talking accelerated ageing, increased fine lines and reduced skin elasticity.

And here's where stress shows its sneaky side. Remember that alarm system we talked about? When it's constantly activated, it triggers inflammation throughout your body. This isn't the helpful kind of inflammation that heals a cut or fights an infection, this is your body's defence system stuck in overdrive, causing collateral damage to healthy tissues. Everything becomes amplified – skin sensitivities increase, healing slows down and age-related changes accelerate. That persistent redness or those stubborn dark circles under your eyes? They might be telling you it's time to address your stress levels.

#PersonalTale

Let me share something from my daily clinic life. Every time I see a patient, I always ask how they're doing: How's work? How's the family? How's life treating you? Nine times out of ten, the answer involves stress. Sometimes it's the pressure of hitting deadlines while juggling school runs. Other times it's relationship troubles, teenage dramas or financial worries. The list seems endless.

In today's society, finding someone who *isn't* stressed is as rare as spotting a unicorn in your garden. I honestly think we all put too much pressure on ourselves and juggle too many balls at one time – and I'm no exception!

The truth is, managing stress requires more than just good intentions and the occasional deep breath. While meditation is wonderful (and, yes, we're coming to that), treating stress effectively needs a more comprehensive approach. Think of it like training for a marathon rather than preparing for a quick sprint away from a spider; it takes consistent effort, the right tools and, most importantly, an understanding that everyone's stress management journey looks different. What works for your yoga-loving colleague might not work for you, and that's perfectly fine; it's not about quick fixes or magic solutions, it's about creating a sustainable strategy that works in real life.

The Power of Sleep.

The most underrated yet crucial stress-management tool is often the one we sacrifice first when life gets hectic: sleep. Far from being just a time for rest, sleep serves as your body's essential repair and rejuvenation period. During these precious hours, your skin works the 'night shift', engaging in serious maintenance work that simply can't happen during the day.

At night, your body ramps up the production of growth hormone, a key player in cellular repair, and increases blood flow to the skin. This is when collagen gets replenished, damaged cells are repaired and the effects of daily wear and tear are reversed. On top of that, sleep reduces cortisol levels, giving your skin a much-needed break from inflammation and excess oil production.

Missing out on quality sleep doesn't just leave you feeling groggy, it can accelerate the ageing process and weaken your skin's natural barrier, leaving it looking dull and fatigued. In short, those late nights scrolling or working come at a high cost to your skin and overall health. Prioritising sleep is one of the simplest yet most impactful ways to support your body's natural stress management and repair processes.

Remember, in the wee hours, your skin cells are working overtime. This is when cell regeneration peaks, running up to three times faster than during the day. You basically have an army of microscopic workers rushing to repair the day's damage while you dream. During these crucial hours, your skin is busy creating new cells, producing fresh collagen and repairing UV damage from when you forgot your SPF (we've all been there).

The science behind this nocturnal restoration is fascinating. Your body's production of growth hormone peaks during deep sleep, triggering a cascade of repair processes. Collagen synthesis kicks into high gear and cell turnover accelerates, helping to shed damaged cells and reveal fresher, healthier skin beneath.

During these hours, your skin is also more receptive to active ingredients than at any other time. Blood flow to your skin increases, cell renewal nearly doubles and your skin's natural barrier becomes more permeable. It's like your skin opens up thousands of tiny doorways, ready to accept help from your carefully chosen skincare products.

Your body temperature also plays a crucial role in this process. It naturally drops at night, which signals your skin to start its repair cycle. This is why sleeping in a cool room (around 18°C) isn't just comfortable, it's supporting your skin's natural renewal process.

I always recommend using a silk pillowcase, too. Not only do they reduce friction (preventing sleep creases that can become permanent) but they also help maintain your skin's moisture levels throughout the night. Cotton can draw moisture away from your skin, rather like sleeping on a moisture-wicking towel.

Here's where sleep and stress management become inseparable. When you're stressed, your cortisol levels remain elevated, which can interfere with your skin's repair cycle. Skip sleep altogether and you're essentially cancelling your skin's repair appointment, sending the technicians home before they've finished the job. One night of poor sleep might show up as dark circles and dull skin, but chronic sleep deprivation has more serious consequences: your skin's barrier function becomes compromised, moisture loss increases, and inflammation levels rise.

#PersonalTale

I see this regularly in clinic – patients who pride themselves on 'running on empty' while wondering why their expensive skincare isn't delivering results. The truth is, no amount of luxury cream can compensate for missing this crucial repair time. Those late-night Netflix binges or extra hours at the office might seem productive, but they're essentially borrowing against your skin's future.

#ActionableSteps

It's nearly impossible to drift off to sleep when you're dealing with high stress levels. If your mind is racing with thoughts and flooded with images and visions, you'll likely find yourself tossing and turning all night. To break free from this cycle, it's essential to boost your oxytocin levels and activate your parasympathetic nervous system, which help your body relax. Implementing a proper wind-down routine is essential. Create a calming pre-bedtime ritual to signal to your body that it's time to switch from 'fight or flight' to 'rest and repair'. This might mean:

- A warm bath (the subsequent temperature drop helps trigger sleep).

- Gentle face massage while applying your nighttime skincare (helps reduce muscle tension and aids product absorption).

- No blue light exposure for at least an hour before bed (no last-minute Instagram scrolling).

- Reading or gentle stretching instead of stimulating activities.

- Setting aside 10 to 15 minutes before bed to practise some meditation. Focus on taking a few slow, deep breaths, letting go of the day's stress and allowing your body to unwind.

When you manage your stress levels before bed, you're not just improving your sleep, you're optimising your skin's entire repair cycle. It's a great example of how interconnected our body's systems are: reduce stress, improve sleep, enhance skin repair, look better, feel better, stress less … and the positive cycle continues.

Exercise might feel like the last thing you want to do when stressed, but it really is one of your body's best defence mechanisms against its ageing effects. Exercise basically presses your body's reset button; each session helps clear out stress hormones and trigger the production of molecules that protect your cells from ageing, giving your body a mini holiday, even if your mind is still worrying about that deadline. I'm not talking about training for a marathon; even a fast walk can trigger the release of endorphins (your body's natural stress fighters).

What you eat can either arm you against stress or leave you more vulnerable to its effects. When I'm stressed, my first instinct is to reach for comfort food (preferably a chocolate biscuit), but I've learned that this only adds to the problem. Stress eating typically means choosing foods that increase inflammageing. Think of food as your stress-management buddy; foods rich in omega-3s, antioxidants and B vitamins help your body build resilience against stress, creating a cellular shield against the ageing effects of your daily pressures.

The Social Connection.
Here's a fascinating truth about ageing that might surprise you: your social connections could be as important as your skincare routine.

When we engage in meaningful interactions with others, our bodies produce a remarkable hormone: oxytocin (our own anti-ageing elixir). While you can't bottle it or buy it in a cream, this 'cuddle chemical' might be one of the most powerful anti-ageing tools we have. So, get hugging.

#PersonalTale

I've seen how my patients with strong social connections often show better stress resilience and, interestingly, better skin health, but it was my own experience with my three dogs that really drove this home.

There's nothing quite like being ambushed by a 40 kg Rottweiler who thinks she's a lap dog to boost your oxytocin levels! While ending up on the floor might not be part of my stress-management plan, those puppy cuddles are literally changing my body chemistry for the better. That said, I think Rottweilers are the neediest breed out there!

Oxytocin is your body's natural stress antidote, working behind the scenes to counter the ageing effects of stress hormones like cortisol. While it might sound scientific, the ways to boost it are delightfully simple: meaningful connections, physical touch, acts of kindness and lots of hugging. A proper 20-second cuddle with someone you care about isn't just comforting, it's medicine; that warm feeling you get when sharing dinner and laughter with friends is not just enjoyment, it's your body producing natural stress-fighting chemicals. Even small acts of kindness like helping a stranger or volunteering trigger this powerful hormone's release.

#ActionableSteps

We all need to declutter now and then – not just our homes, but our lives. Sometimes, creating peace isn't about more storage, it's about letting go of what no longer serves us.

Relationships. Have you ever done a relationship reality check? It's worth it. Sift out the people who drain your energy, those friends who leave you exhausted after every call, the relatives who never fail to criticise. It's okay to create boundaries or even cut ties with those who negatively impact your emotional wellbeing. Protecting your inner peace isn't selfish, it's essential.

Digital Detox. Social media, unfortunately, has the tendency to make us feel inadequate. If this is happening, press 'Delete'. Are Insta news feeds keeping you awake at night? Delete. Your phone should be a tool not a source of stress. Taking control of your digital world is an act of self-care.

Financial Freedom. Sometimes, what we call an investment turns out to be more of a burden, whether it's an overstretched property, a barely used subscription or, in my case, a piece of art that's *supposed* to appreciate in value someday. Letting go of these commitments can be incredibly freeing. True financial freedom isn't just about earning more, it's about understanding that less can often mean so much more.

Career Clarity. Are you living to work or working to live? If your job is leaving you drained, it's not just impacting your stress levels, it's taking a toll on your health. Recognising when something isn't right and having the courage to make a change can be one of the most empowering and transformative decisions you'll ever make.

Calendar Control. My husband is the king of back-to-back meetings, but even he's learning that scheduled breaks are as vital as the meetings themselves. Time to decompress isn't a luxury, it's a necessity. Give yourself space to think and breathe.

The Power of 'No'. I'll admit, this one hits close to home – I'm still learning it myself. Every time you agree to something you'd rather avoid, you're giving up time and energy that could be spent on something you truly enjoy. Start practising saying no – it's a skill that gets easier with time, I promise.

Delegation. Are you shouldering tasks that aren't truly yours? It's time to pass them back. Supporting others doesn't mean taking on every burden. Learning to say 'This isn't my responsibility' can be incredibly liberating.

Reducing stressors isn't selfish, it's essential. You wouldn't keep pouring water into an already overflowing cup, so don't keep adding pressure to an overloaded life. Clear the clutter, let go and make room for what truly matters. Reduced stress = reduced ageing.

#DrVixTakeaways
It's not realistic to think we can spend every moment meditating, exercising, eating healthily, getting quality sleep and cutting out

alcohol. Life is busy, and balance is key! After decades in aesthetic medicine and managing my own stress responses (including notorious spider encounters), here's what really matters:

1. Stress isn't your enemy, it's your ancient survival system needing an update. Don't try to eliminate it, learn to reset it.

2. Sleep is non-negotiable. If you only change one thing, make it sleep. It's your body's most powerful anti-ageing program and it's free.

3. Your stressed body processes food differently. Choose anti-inflammatory foods when under pressure – your cells will thank you.

4. Movement trumps motivation. Forget 'perfect' exercise, just move in ways you enjoy. Consistency beats intensity every time.

5. Master the two-minute reset. When stress hits, take two minutes to focus solely on breathing. It's not meditation, it's rewiring your stress response. You can't control all stressors, but you can control your response. Each time you choose a conscious response over a reactive one, you're resetting your biological age.

CHAPTER 10:
PILLOW TALK

Your Nighttime Cellular Repair

When was the last time you could honestly say you had a truly good night's sleep – one where you didn't wake up every hour to head to the loo or lie there staring at the ceiling while your mind races with a never-ending list of tasks, worries and unfinished thoughts? A night after which you actually felt refreshed and ready to take on the day instead of feeling drained and foggy? If that sounds like a rarity, you're definitely not alone. Many of us struggle to get that kind of deep, restorative sleep, and it's a bigger issue than we might realise.

I experienced the devastating effects of sleep deprivation first-hand during my years as a junior doctor. Yes, that was nearly 30 years ago! Working 36-hour shifts with barely any rest, like many doctors in that era, we were expected to make life-changing medical decisions while our cognitive function was severely compromised. How could any of us possibly make sound judgements in that state? I remember trying to calculate medication dosages at 3 a.m. after being awake for nearly 30 hours, my brain feeling like it was wading through treacle. Thankfully, regulations for junior doctors have now changed significantly, making medicine safer for both healthcare providers and patients alike, but those experiences gave me a profound appreciation for how critical proper sleep is for cognitive function.

I know we touched on sleep in the last chapter, but I'm dedicating this entire chapter to sleep because it truly is vital to your health and wellbeing. It's intricately linked to our physical health, mental clarity and emotional resilience. Yet, for many, achieving a good night's kip can feel like an elusive goal, especially in the face of life's daily challenges.

#PersonalTale
Sleep is my ultimate sanctuary, my be-all and end-all, especially if I'm injecting patients the next day! However, my pursuit of a peaceful night is often interrupted by unmistakable nocturnal sounds …

After years of 'acoustic challenges' (wink wink), I've engineered what I call my 'sleep sanctuary'. Picture this: I'm lying there like some sci-fi sleep warrior, complete with an eye mask and 'Princess Leia headphones', blocking out all nighttime noises. Not exactly the romantic setup from *The Notebook*, and yes, I probably look utterly ridiculous, but between looking silly and being a sleep-deprived zombie the next day, I'll take silly every time.

Sometimes the best solutions aren't the prettiest, but a well-rested me is a happy me!

Sleep is your body's nightly restoration program, going far beyond just waking up feeling refreshed. It's a complex biological process that impacts numerous functions from cellular repair to inflammation regulation. While you sleep, your body carries out essential tasks that promote physical recovery, cognitive function and emotional balance. Yet, in today's fast-paced world, quality sleep has become harder to come by. Unfortunately, sleep is often the first thing we sacrifice to improve productivity, trading precious restoration time for one more email, one more episode or one more scroll through social media, without realising we're making withdrawals from our health accounts that no amount of caffeine can repay.

From what I've heard from both patients and friends, sleep has become a real struggle for many since the arrival of COVID-19. The pandemic threw a curveball into our routines, bringing a host of stressors that dramatically reshaped our lives. As a result, sleep often took a backseat, leading to a surge in insomnia and restless nights. COVID-19 became the ultimate 'inflammager', not only affecting us on a viral level but ramping up inflammation throughout the body, creating a vicious cycle where poor sleep fuels inflammation, and inflammation, in turn, makes sleep even harder to come by.

The Circadian Rhythm.

Your circadian rhythm is your body's internal clock that follows a 24-hour cycle, regulating key processes like sleep, hormone production and metabolism. This natural rhythm is closely tied to the light-dark cycle in the environment, syncing with the rising and setting of the sun.

When your circadian rhythm is in sync, it maximises energy, focus and recovery, helping you feel alert during the day and restful at night. However, when this delicate balance is disrupted – whether from irregular sleep patterns, shift work or too much exposure to artificial light – it can have a serious impact on your health, affecting everything from mood to immune function.

Taking care of your circadian rhythm is essential for improving sleep, boosting wellbeing and living a more vibrant life. Let's take a look at how it works:

Early Morning (4–6 a.m.). As dawn breaks, cortisol levels start to rise, preparing your body for waking. This 'cortisol awakening response' is essential. It promotes alertness, regulates blood pressure and mobilises your energy reserves. Most of us are blissfully unaware of what is going on here.

Morning (6–9 a.m.). Cortisol peaks during these hours, while melatonin production comes to a halt. Thyroid levels rise, and your body temperature begins to climb. This natural rise in energy explains why morning exercise feels particularly invigorating – your body is primed for activity, ready to take on the world.

Mid-morning to Early Afternoon (10 a.m.–2 p.m.). Here, you'll find yourself at the height of alertness. Your coordination is sharp, cognitive performance is optimal, and your metabolism is firing on all cylinders. It's the time of day when you're most equipped to tackle complex tasks and challenges and get through those emails!

Afternoon (2–6 p.m.). As the day wears on, you might notice the infamous afternoon slump. Your chocolate biscuit cravings kick-in and you could easily have a power kip. Your alertness declines and cortisol levels begin to drop, signalling that your body is ready for a brief reprieve. Sound familiar?

Evening (6–10 p.m.). As the sun sets, your body temperature starts to cool and melatonin production begins to rise, preparing you for rest. Metabolism slows and cortisol levels continue to fall, ushering in a sense of calm. This transition into evening is critical for winding down and letting go of the day's stressors.

Night (10 p.m.–2 a.m.). This period marks a vital window for your body's repair processes. Here, growth hormone levels peak, melatonin reaches its highest levels and cellular repair is maximised. Your skin undergoes its most effective regeneration and your immune system works at its strongest, fighting off potential threats. So, this timeframe is your anti-ageing friend.

Early Morning (2–4 a.m.). In the depths of the night, you enter the deepest sleep phase. Your body temperature is at its lowest and tissue repair is most intense, allowing your body to heal and rejuvenate itself thoroughly.

CIRCADIAN RHYTHM

Early Morning (4-6 AM)

At dawn, cortisol rises, waking your body and boosting alertness, blood pressure, and energy. This essential 'Cortisol Awakening Response' happens unnoticed by most of us.

Morning boosts: Cortisol peaks, melatonin halts, thyroid hormones rise, and body temperature climbs - priming you for energising workouts and a productive day.

Morning (6-9 AM)

Mid-Morning to Early Afternoon (10 AM-2 PM)

This is your peak: sharp coordination, optimal cognitive performance, and high metabolism - perfect for tackling complex tasks.

As the day goes on, the afternoon slump hits: cravings kick in, alertness dips, and cortisol drops - your body's cue for a quick recharge.

Afternoon (2-6 PM)

Evening (6-10 PM)

As evening sets in, your body cools, melatonin rises, and cortisol falls - preparing you to relax, unwind, and rest.

This is your body's repair peak: growth hormones surge, melatonin is highest, cells regenerate, and immunity strengthens - your ultimate anti-ageing window.

Night (10 PM-2 AM)

Early Morning (2-4 AM)

In the depths of the night, you enter the deepest sleep phase. Your body temperature is at its lowest, and tissue repair is most intense, allowing your body to heal and rejuvenate itself thoroughly.

Your Circadian Rhythm

Understanding this rhythm is crucial, especially as modern life often forces us to work against it. When we indulge in late-night binge eating after a night out, we are asking our digestive systems to work during their natural downtime. When we expose ourselves to bright screens in the evenings (mainly from our phones, laptops and TVs), we confuse our melatonin production, throwing our rhythms into disarray. Shift work and travel across time zones are also common disruptors to our sleep patterns.

Each of these creates a cascade of effects throughout your system, potentially accelerating the ageing process through heightened inflammation and disrupted repair cycles. Poor sleep isn't just about dark circles under your eyes; even one night of disrupted sleep increases inflammatory markers throughout your body. Studies show that sleep-deprived individuals show higher levels of inflammatory mediators (key players in chronic inflammation).

#ActionableSteps

We need to go beyond basic sleep hygiene measures here. While you've probably heard the usual advice about dark rooms and regular bedtimes, optimising sleep requires a more comprehensive approach.

The Timing Factor. Your body's production of cortisol and melatonin are tightly regulated by consistent signals from your environment. One of the most powerful cues to help set your circadian rhythm is exposure to natural sunlight, particularly in the morning. Getting outside within an hour of waking helps kickstart your day by signalling to your body that it's time to be awake and alert.

On the flip side, exposure to artificial light, especially blue light from your phone and laptop, can interfere with your natural sleep signals by suppressing melatonin production. This can leave you feeling wide awake at bedtime, making it harder to wind down and get a good night's sleep. So, if you're hoping for better rest, it's a good idea to ditch the Instagram feed.

Temperature Regulation. Did you know that your body temperature needs to drop for optimal sleep. A cool room (around

18°C) supports this natural decline. However, cold feet can disrupt sleep!

Supplementation.

While improving sleep habits is fundamental, sometimes our bodies need additional support. Through years of clinical practice, I've found certain supplements particularly effective when used correctly, and no, they are not all prescribed medications, which tend to be addictive.

Melatonin. One of my favourite supplements as a short-term kick. But here's what most people don't realise: it's not just your sleep buddy, it's actually one of your body's most powerful natural anti-inflammatory compounds.

The trick is timing it right, and I see so many of my patients getting this wrong, popping tablets like sweets, thinking more is better. It's not. Remember, we're trying to whisper to your body's natural rhythm, not shout at it. Always start small – just 3 mg about 2 hours before you want to drift off. Why 2 hours? Because you're mimicking your body's natural melatonin release pattern. Take it too late and you'll wake up feeling like you're wearing a lead blanket; take it too early and you might miss your sleep window entirely.

Ashwagandha. Another favourite of mine that has emerged as a key player in sleep optimisation. This adaptogenic herb helps regulate cortisol levels, making it particularly useful for those whose racing minds keep them awake. It works best when taken consistently, not just on sleepless nights.

Magnesium. Your nervous system's natural tranquiliser, orchestrating calm throughout your body. This essential mineral plays a crucial role in over 300 biochemical reactions, but its relationship with GABA (gamma-aminobutyric acid) is particularly fascinating. GABA is your brain's primary inhibitory neurotransmitter, essentially working as your neural brake pedal, slowing down the constant firing of stress signals. Magnesium supports GABA production. Many of us are magnesium deficient, and supplementation often improves not just sleep quality but also muscle relaxation and stress resilience.

When magnesium levels drop in our stressed, chaotic lives, a cascade of effects follows, impacting muscle tension, sleep quality and our ability to handle stress. Without adequate magnesium, your nervous system loses its natural dampeners, making everything feel more intense and overwhelming. This creates a challenging cycle: stress depletes magnesium, low magnesium reduces stress resilience.

Modern diets, high in processed foods and grown in depleted soils, compound the problem by providing less magnesium than our bodies need. Breaking this cycle through supplementation can have profound effects. While subtle at first, restoring optimal magnesium levels helps rebalance your nervous system's natural ability to find calm. People often report deeper sleep, better emotional balance, and improved stress handling – not through sedation, but through supporting their body's innate capacity for resilience.

Glycine. An amino acid that acts as both a neurotransmitter and a building block for protein, playing an interesting dual role in sleep regulation. When you consume glycine-rich foods – like bone broth, collagen or gelatine – you're not just supporting skin health, you're providing your brain with a powerful sleep-enhancing compound. Glycine lowers your core body temperature, which signals your brain that it's time for sleep, while simultaneously calming your nervous system.

Tryptophan. Melatonin's amino acid precursor; the raw material your body needs to manufacture your natural sleep hormone.

However, timing and food combining are crucial for effective use of amino acid supplements. Tryptophan needs help crossing the blood-brain barrier. Complex carbohydrates – such as quinoa, sweet potato and oats – trigger insulin release, which clears competing amino acids from your bloodstream, creating a clearer path for tryptophan to reach your brain. Eating glycine and tryptophan too close to bedtime can disrupt sleep by triggering digestion. Instead, including glycine-rich foods and tryptophan-carbohydrate combinations at dinner, ideally three to four hours before bed, allows your body to process these nutrients optimally. For those struggling with morning grogginess, the glycine connection is particularly relevant as it helps regulate your core temperature rhythm, often leading to more refreshing sleep and clearer mornings.

Regular consumption of these sleep-supporting nutrients can help reset disrupted sleep patterns over time, working with your body's natural rhythm rather than forcing sleep through artificial means.

So, we have discovered that sleep disruption creates a vicious cycle with hormone imbalance. Poor sleep elevates cortisol, which, in turn, makes quality sleep more difficult. Meanwhile, growth hormone – crucial for repair and regeneration – is primarily released during deep sleep phases.

This relationship becomes particularly relevant during menopause and andropause, when hormonal changes often disrupt sleep patterns. Supporting sleep during these transitions isn't just about feeling better, it's about maintaining your body's repair mechanisms.

Your Biochemical Schedule.

After years in GP land helping patients optimise their sleep and witnessing its profound effects on ageing, I've learned that quality sleep is about working with your body's natural rhythms, not against them.

We all have a natural sleep blueprint, and understanding your chronotype – whether you're naturally an early bird or night owl – is crucial for healthy ageing. Fighting your natural rhythm is like swimming against the current; it creates unnecessary stress on your body. If you're most productive at night, don't force yourself into a 5 a.m. workout routine just because it's trending. (I'm definitely an early bird and like to be tucked up by 10 p.m. for me to function!)

Consistency is also paramount; your body craves routine more than perfection. A consistent seven hours of sleep delivers better results than alternating between five and nine hours. Think of it like nutrition – regular, balanced patterns win over erratic cycles. Aim to keep your sleep and wake times within a one-hour window, even on weekends.

Understanding your body's biochemical schedule can also transform your sleep quality. Think of your day as a series of crucial timing decisions, each affecting how well you'll sleep later. That afternoon coffee you rely on? Its effects linger far longer than you might expect, which is why I recommend making 2 p.m. your caffeine cutoff time. Similarly, while exercise is excellent for sleep, intense workouts too close to bedtime can leave your body too energised to rest. Aim to finish vigorous activity at least three hours before bed.

The timing of your evening meal is equally crucial. Finishing your supper three hours before sleep gives your digestive system time to settle, allowing your body to focus on repair and restoration rather than processing food. Even supplement timing matters – some energise, while others promote relaxation, so when you take them can make a significant difference.

But how do you know if you're getting it right?

Your body sends clear signals about sleep quality. That morning glow (or lack thereof) isn't just about beauty, it's one of your body's most visible sleep quality indicators. Watch for other signs, too: how quickly you recover from exercise, your emotional balance throughout the day and your energy stability. These aren't just random benefits, they're your body's way of communicating whether your sleep is truly restorative.

Remember: your sleep is not self-indulgence, it's self-preservation. Everything from skin repair to cellular regeneration and hormone balance to inflammation control relies on quality sleep. By prioritising sleep, you're investing not only in tomorrow's energy but in your long-term health and longevity.

#DrVixTakeaways

1. Your circadian rhythm is more than just a sleep-wake cycle, it's your body's 24-hour master clock. Those precious hours between 10 p.m. and 2 a.m. are your skin's anti-ageing sweet spot, when cellular repair and growth hormone production

peak. Miss this window regularly and you're skipping your body's natural beauty treatment.

2. Sleep disruption is an 'inflammager' – even one bad night increases inflammatory markers throughout your body. Poor sleep accelerates ageing from the inside out by disrupting your body's repair mechanisms.

3. A 90-minute wind-down before bed is crucial. Like a computer, your brain needs time to properly 'shut down' – dimming lights, reducing blue light exposure and regulating temperature all signal to your body that it's time for sleep.

4. Supplementation needs to be strategic. More isn't always better. Start with small doses of melatonin (1–2 mg), consider magnesium and time your nutrients right. Remember: the goal isn't to knock yourself out but to support your natural sleep rhythm.

5. Temperature matters more than you think. Aim for 18°C in your bedroom but keep your feet warm. And if you need to wear 'Princess Leia headphones' and an eye mask, like I do, embrace it! Sometimes the least romantic solution is the most effective.

CHAPTER 11:
CONTROL + ALT + REJUVENATE

The Future Is Biohacking

If someone had told me 20 years ago that we'd be using data science to hack our biology for better skin and slower ageing, I'd have thought they'd been watching too much sci-fi. Yet, here we are – tracking blood sugar in real time, measuring sleep architecture with smart rings and running lab tests from our living rooms.

Welcome to biohacking, where science meets self-optimisation and your body becomes your most fascinating experiment. While new clinics are offering high-tech treatments with equally high-tech price tags, some of the most powerful biological optimisations can happen right at home. I'm talking about science-backed tweaks like strategic cold exposure (that final 30 seconds of cold shower I'm still working up the courage to try!), targeted supplement timing and precision light exposure.

The best part? You don't need a PhD to join in. That afternoon energy crash you blame on poor willpower? Your glucose monitor might reveal it's actually a blood sugar rollercoaster triggered by your 'healthy' lunch. Those bouts of brain fog? Your sleep tracker might show breathing disruptions fragmenting your deep sleep.

Biohacking isn't about becoming a cyborg, it's about gathering personal data, running small experiments and discovering what works for your unique biology. It rejects one-size-fits-all advice that treats us as statistics rather than individuals with distinct genetic blueprints and hormonal patterns.

This chapter cuts through the hype to focus on evidence-based approaches that deliver measurable results without requiring a second mortgage or a biochemistry degree. Your body is the most sophisticated technology you'll ever own – biohacking just helps you read the manual better.

Think of biohacking as becoming the CEO of your own biology. Instead of blindly following generic health advice or hoping that expensive cream will work magic, biohackers take a data-driven approach to optimisation. We're not just talking about tracking steps or counting calories, this is about understanding everything from your sleep cycles to your cellular health, your stress responses to your skin's repair mechanisms. It's like having a dashboard for your body, where every metric can be measured, monitored and improved.

You know how everyone tells you either that coffee is good or bad for you? Well, biohacking can show exactly how *your* body responds to your early morning cappuccino, revealing exactly how it affects your blood sugar. And your sleep? It might just explain why you're still exhausted despite getting your 'eight hours'.

The beauty of biohacking lies in its precision. After years in both traditional medicine and aesthetics, I find this absolutely fascinating. Instead of relying on one-size-fits-all health advice (the kind that seems to change every week in the media), we can now see exactly what works for each individual, gathering real data about how your own body responds to different interventions.

Biohacking takes everything we know about ageing and turns it into actionable data. In clinic, I often see patients who are doing everything 'right' – prescription skincare, regular treatments – but still not getting optimal results. Often, the missing piece is understanding their internal inflammation levels. Biohacking tools like continuous glucose monitors, sleep trackers and inflammatory markers testing can reveal what's really going on beneath the surface.

Let's break down some practical biohacking approaches that I've seen work wonders. First: sleep. It's not just about getting eight hours, it's about optimising your sleep environment. Temperature, light exposure and sleep timing all affect your skin's repair processes. I've seen patients' skin transform simply by adjusting their sleep environment to optimise their circadian rhythm.

Next up: diet. Modern biohacking has revolutionised our understanding of nutrition by revealing it's profoundly individual. Through continuous glucose monitoring and other testing, my patients have made eye-opening discoveries: foods traditionally recommended as nutritious were secretly triggering dramatic blood sugar fluctuations, causing insulin surges and igniting inflammatory responses. Many found that their morning bowl of wholegrain cereal created more metabolic chaos than a simple protein-rich breakfast of avocado and eggs. These personalised insights often contradict popular recommendations but deliver remarkable results when you respond to your body's actual data rather than following generic advice.

#PersonalTale

Recently, I signed up for ZOE, a personalised nutrition app. It provides tailored insights into how my body responds to food by monitoring factors like blood sugar, blood fat and gut health.

The program sent me a kit with a blood sugar monitor, a blood fat test, a stool sample kit and specific foods to help test gut transit time. Based on this data, it tracked how different foods impacted my body and offered guidance on dietary adjustments to reduce inflammation and support overall health. Now, I regularly scan what I eat (within reason) to keep an eye on my weight and better understand how my body responds to certain foods – particularly what might trigger blood sugar spikes or lead to fat storage. More on this later.

NAD+.

Another hot topic in anti-ageing science currently is nicotinamide adenine dinucleotide (NAD+). This remarkable molecule (whose full name is quite a mouthful!) is present in every cell of your body, quietly modulating the ageing process behind the scenes. Don't worry if you've never heard of it, just think of it as your cells' rechargeable battery. Just as your phone needs charging to function, every single cell in your body needs NAD+ to produce energy, repair DNA and keep you feeling young and vibrant.

Why is NAD+ so crucial? First, it's your cells' energy currency converter, transforming the food you eat into ATP (adenosine tri-phosphate), the fuel your cells actually use. It is also your cellular repair crew, fixing damaged DNA and supporting special proteins called sirtuins that help keep your cells young and healthy.

When we're young, our NAD+ levels are high – it's why children seem to have endless energy and bounce back from injuries so quickly – but by the time we hit 50, these levels have plummeted to about half of what they were, leading to less energy, slower recovery and accelerated ageing.

The exciting part? Scientists have discovered that we can actually boost our NAD+ levels through specific lifestyle changes and targeted supplements. We can recharge our body's cellular batteries! This is why it has become such a hot topic in anti-ageing medicine. By maintaining healthy NAD+ levels, we might be able to keep our cellular batteries charged, potentially slowing down the ageing process and maintaining our vitality longer.

Temperature as Medicine: Hot and Cold Therapies for Longevity.

Living in the New Forest, I watch my friends brave the Solent's chilly waters between the mainland and the Isle of Wight, even during the winter months. They are nuts! While I prefer my water at a more comfortable temperature, the science behind temperature exposure – both cold and heat – is becoming harder to ignore.

Let's start with cold therapy, which gained mainstream popularity through Wim Hof, nicknamed 'The Iceman'. He transformed cold exposure from an eccentric practice into a scientifically studied longevity tool. Through remarkable feats like climbing Mount Everest in shorts and maintaining his core temperature in ice baths, he's demonstrated how cold exposure can change our understanding of human potential.

What happens when you immerse yourself in cold water goes far beyond the initial shock, gasping breaths and goosebumps! Your body initiates a cascade of biological responses. This controlled stress, what scientists call 'hormesis', is like sending your cells to boot camp – they emerge stronger and more resilient. Cold exposure triggers the production of brown fat (the good kind that helps burn the white fat we're typically trying to lose) and activates a powerful anti-inflammatory response.

The beauty of cold exposure is that you don't need to swim in the winter Solent to benefit (though my brave friends might disagree). Even a 30-second cold shower at the end of your regular shower can stimulate these longevity pathways. It's about creating controlled stress that makes your body more resilient.

Interestingly, while cold therapy works wonders for many people, emerging research suggests that women might actually benefit more from heat-based therapies like saunas. Recent studies indicate that women's hormonal profiles respond differently to temperature extremes, with sauna use showing particularly promising effects on female longevity markers, cardiovascular health and stress resilience. This gender difference might explain why I've always intuitively preferred hot baths to cold plunges!

The Finnish have long understood the health benefits of sauna bathing, with regular users showing significantly lower rates of cardiovascular disease, dementia and all-cause mortality. The heat stress activates heat-shock proteins that help repair damaged cells, improves vascular function and increases growth hormone production – all particularly beneficial during perimenopause and beyond.

For women specifically, regular sauna sessions (2–3 times weekly) have been linked to more balanced cortisol patterns, improved sleep quality and reduced inflammation – three factors that profoundly impact both skin health and ageing. The increased circulation brings nutrient-rich blood to the skin's surface, potentially delivering better results than many expensive topical treatments.

What's fascinating is that both hot and cold therapies work through similar hormetic mechanisms – controlled stress that triggers adaptive responses – but they activate slightly different pathways, making them complementary rather than competitive approaches.

So, whether you're drawn to cold plunges or hot saunas (I know which camp I'm in!), the evidence supports temperature as a powerful biohacking tool. Personally, I'm working up the courage to end my shower with just 15 seconds of cold water while enjoying regular sauna sessions – starting small with temperature contrast therapy seems like a reasonable compromise even for cold-averse people like me!

Red-Light Therapy.

This is a treatment we frequently use in the clinic, both before and after procedures.

Understanding how different types of light impact skin and cellular health is essential. We're all aware of the need to limit UV exposure to prevent skin damage, but red-light therapy has unique, beneficial effects. When applied in controlled sessions, red light penetrates deeply into the skin, where it stimulates collagen production, aiding in skin firmness and elasticity. It also has powerful anti-inflammatory effects, reducing redness and swelling, supporting healing and promoting an overall healthier complexion.

All this makes red-light therapy an effective, non-invasive option for boosting skin health and enhancing treatment results.

The Blue Zone Blueprint.

This is the fascinating discovery where ancient wisdom meets modern science. Did you know, there are regions in the world where people routinely live past 100 in remarkably good health? These 'Blue Zones', discovered by researcher Dan Buettner, offer living proof that extended vitality isn't just about genetics, it's about lifestyle.

From Okinawa to Sardinia, the Greek island of Ikaria to Costa Rica's Nicoya Peninsula, and even in Loma Linda, California, communities have been unknowingly 'biohacking' their way to longevity for generations. Modern science is now validating what these people have always known instinctively, and it turns out their 'secrets' aren't actually secrets at all, they're simple, daily practises that have profound effects.

Let's explore what makes these Blue Zone populations thrive. Take their approach to social connection. While we're glued to our phones, these communities prioritise real human interaction. They gather for meals, celebrate together and support each other through life's challenges. This constant face-to-face social engagement naturally boosts oxytocin (our feel-good hormone) and reduces stress – no meditation app required!

Movement looks different in these regions, too. You won't find fancy gyms or high-intensity boot camps. Instead, physical activity is woven into the fabric of daily life – walking to visit friends, tending gardens or dancing at community gatherings. It's constant, gentle movement rather than sporadic, intense exercise.

Their eating patterns are particularly interesting, naturally following what we now tout as the latest dietary trends. Their plates are filled with plant-based foods rich in natural anti-inflammatory compounds, and they practise regular fasting periods – though they wouldn't call it 'intermittent fasting', it's simply part of their cultural or religious practices.

#PersonalTale

What strikes me most is how these communities achieve extraordinary health outcomes through ordinary practices. While we're tracking steps and counting macros, they're simply living in ways that naturally promote longevity. Perhaps that's the real secret: making healthy choices so routine they don't require conscious effort.

The beauty of these findings? Every single one of these longevity practices can be adapted to our modern lives. We don't need to move to Okinawa, we just need to understand and apply these time-tested principles in our own context.

Metformin.

While Blue Zone populations naturally maintain low inflammation through lifestyle choices, modern medicine has discovered a fascinating parallel – medications that similarly help control inflammation might offer some of the same longevity benefits. One particularly intriguing candidate emerging from this research is metformin, a well-established diabetes medication with an unexpected story.

The scientific interest in metformin's potential anti-ageing properties began with a remarkable observation: diabetic patients taking metformin often had longer lifespans than non-diabetic individuals. This unexpected finding led researchers to look more closely at how this medication might influence the fundamental processes of ageing.

At its core, metformin works like a cellular efficiency expert. It activates a powerful molecule called adenosine monophosphate-activated protein kinase (AMPK), which acts as your body's energy manager. When AMPK is activated, it turns on your cells' housekeeping service, cleaning up cellular debris, managing energy use more efficiently and keeping inflammation in check.

However, metformin's influence on inflammation might be its most remarkable feature. As we've discussed throughout this book, chronic inflammation accelerates ageing across all body systems. Metformin acts like a careful conductor, helping to quiet the inflammatory orchestra without silencing it completely. It doesn't suppress inflammation like steroids do; instead, it helps regulate the inflammatory response to a more youthful level.

Metformin has a powerful connection with insulin, and its relationship with ageing is remarkably close. Imagine insulin as the key that unlocks your cells, allowing glucose to enter. Over time, these 'locks' can start to rust, requiring more and more insulin to function properly. Metformin works to keep these locks well oiled, helping to maintain your cells' sensitivity to insulin. And it's not just about blood sugar, improved insulin sensitivity means more efficient energy use, reduced inflammation and a slower ageing process overall.

Now this is possibly the most intriguing connection: metformin's potential role in cancer prevention. Research suggests that people taking metformin have lower rates of various cancers, perhaps because it helps regulate cellular energy production and growth. Cancer cells are energy gluttons, consuming glucose at high rates. Metformin appears to make this feast more difficult, potentially helping to prevent cancer cell growth before it starts. Fascinating, heh?

Lastly, your gut microbiome – that vast community of bacteria living in your intestines – which plays a crucial role in ageing, appears to be beneficially reshaped by metformin. Like having a skilled gardener tending to your internal ecosystem, metformin promotes the growth of beneficial bacteria while weeding out the troublemakers. This influence on gut bacteria might explain many of metformin's benefits beyond blood sugar control. A healthier gut microbiome means better nutrient absorption, stronger immune function and more balanced inflammation levels throughout the body.

Another thing that makes metformin particularly remarkable is how these benefits work together. Each effect reinforces the others, creating a virtuous cycle that supports healthy ageing. The AMPK activation leads to better energy utilisation, which improves insulin sensitivity, which reduces inflammation, which supports a healthy gut microbiome, which further reduces inflammation – and the cycle continues.

However, it's crucial to note that while this research is promising, metformin is still primarily a diabetes medication. Any use for ageing-related purposes should be discussed with healthcare providers, as individual responses and appropriateness can vary significantly. The scientific community continues to study metformin's potential role in ageing, but much research remains to be done.

While metformin has taken centre stage, it's not alone in the longevity medicine cabinet. Scientists are exploring several promising compounds that might help us age better.

What makes these medications particularly interesting is their ability to influence our cells' basic ageing mechanisms. Rather than just treating the symptoms of ageing, they appear to affect the ageing process itself, like adjusting your body's biological software rather than just dealing with hardware problems as they arise.

Low-dose naltrexone. Originally used for addiction treatment, researchers noticed it had unexpected anti-inflammatory and immune-modulating properties. At tiny doses, it appears to help regulate the body's immune response and reduce chronic inflammation.

GLP-1 and GIP Agonists: Metabolism Drugs with Anti-Ageing Potential.

Next up are the glucagon-like peptide-1 (GLP-1) and glucose-dependent insulinotropic polypeptide (GIP) agonists – currently the most talked about compounds in metabolic medicine. You've undoubtedly heard the buzz about Mounjaro, Ozempic, Wegovy and similar medications – they've dominated headlines, sparked social media debates and possibly even come up in conversations with friends experiencing dramatic transformations – but behind the celebrity endorsements and TikTok trends lies fascinating science with implications far beyond just weight loss. Scientists have discovered that these hormones controlling hunger and metabolism might hold keys to longevity that extend far beyond weight management.

Let me break down exactly how these exciting drugs work:

When you consume food, specialised cells in your intestines naturally release GLP-1 and GIP. These hormones orchestrate a sophisticated metabolic response: signalling your pancreas to release insulin (only when blood sugar is elevated), slowing gastric emptying to prolong fullness and communicating with your brain's satiety centres to reduce hunger.

These medications are clever 'enhanced versions' of these natural hormones. They bind to the same receptors but with two crucial advantages: they resist enzymatic breakdown that would normally quickly degrade natural hormones, and they're engineered to stimulate these pathways more potently.

When activating GLP-1 receptors in your brain's hypothalamus, they reduce appetite signals and increase satiety. Simultaneously, in your pancreas, they enhance insulin release only when blood glucose is elevated. The addition of GIP activation in newer dual agonists creates a synergistic effect – GIP enhances GLP-1's action while having independent beneficial effects on fat metabolism.

What's truly fascinating is the cascade of effects beyond appetite and blood sugar control. They appear to fundamentally shift metabolic programming by:

- Reducing systemic inflammation through decreased production of pro-inflammatory cytokines

- Improving mitochondrial function, essentially upgrading your cellular 'batteries'

- Enhancing autophagy – your cells' crucial cleanup and recycling process

- Positively impacting the gut microbiome, potentially resetting problematic bacterial patterns.

During clinical trials, researchers noticed patients weren't just losing weight, they were showing improvements in multiple markers of ageing. Cardiovascular risk factors improved dramatically, cognitive function enhanced and inflammatory markers decreased significantly. These effects occurred even with modest weight loss, suggesting mechanisms beyond simple weight reduction.

What makes these compounds particularly interesting from a biohacking perspective is that they mimic metabolic benefits typically associated with fasting and caloric restriction – long considered gold-standard interventions for longevity – without requiring the same dietary discipline. They essentially 'trick' your body into a metabolically advantageous state.

They appear to work at the root cause, addressing multiple aspects of metabolic health, showing that the connections between metabolism, ageing and overall health are far more intertwined than previously thought. This represents a significant shift in medical thinking – moving from treating individual symptoms to addressing underlying metabolic processes.

Remember our ongoing discussion about inflammation being at the heart of ageing? These medications break the cycle of metabolic inflammation. When patients lose weight with these drugs, they're not just dropping pounds, they're reducing their body's entire inflammatory burden.

#PersonalTale

In practice, I've seen remarkable transformations in patients using these medications. Even personally, I not only lost significant weight but saw improvements in my skin quality, energy levels and inflammatory markers, and was definitely less achy.

However – and this is crucial – these medications aren't magical solutions. They are sophisticated tools that can *enhance* an already healthy lifestyle, not *replace* it. The foundation of healthy ageing still rests on the basics: good nutrition, regular exercise, quality sleep and stress management. Medications can amplify these efforts but cannot compensate for poor lifestyle choices.

One last hack…

Auricular Vagal Neuromodulation Therapy: The Next Frontier in Nervous System Biohacking.

Since we've explored various biohacking approaches throughout this chapter, it's worth examining one of the most promising emerging technologies in the field: Auricular Vagal Neuromodulation Therapy (AVNT). This approach represents the intersection of ancient knowledge about the body's neural pathways and cutting-edge technology designed to access them non-invasively.

The Vagus Nerve: Your Body's Master Regulator.

The vagus nerve – whose name derives from the Latin word for 'wandering' – is arguably your body's most fascinating neural highway. As your longest cranial nerve, it serves as the primary communication pathway between your brain and major organs, including your heart, lungs and digestive system. This explains why it plays such a critical role in regulating inflammation, stress responses and even mood.

Traditional biohacking approaches we've discussed – cold exposure, meditation, breathwork – all indirectly stimulate the vagus nerve. However, modern neuromodulation technology now offers a more direct approach through devices designed specifically to target this crucial nerve through the ear.

How AVNT Works.

Auricular Vagal Neuromodulation Therapy delivers carefully calibrated micro-current electrical impulses to specific points on the ear (typically the tragus) where branches of the vagus nerve are accessible just beneath the skin. When these impulses reach the brainstem, they trigger a cascade of responses that can significantly impact both autonomic nervous system function and inflammatory pathways.

What makes this approach particularly fascinating from a biohacking perspective is its precision. Unlike more diffuse techniques like cold plunges or breathwork (which certainly have their place), AVNT targets the vagus nerve directly, potentially offering more consistent and measurable outcomes.

The Inflammation-Energy Connection.

One of the most compelling applications of AVNT relates directly to our discussions about the relationship between inflammation and energy production. As we've seen throughout this book, chronic inflammation creates a persistent drain on cellular energy, contributing to fatigue and accelerated ageing.

Current research suggests that vagal nerve stimulation may help break this cycle by activating what scientists call the 'cholinergic anti-inflammatory pathway' – a neural mechanism that directly suppresses the production of inflammatory cytokines. By reducing this inflammatory burden, more cellular resources become available for energy production and repair.

This may explain why some users report significant improvements in energy levels and recovery after using these devices consistently. By dampening the inflammatory response, the body can redirect resources from constant immune system activation toward cellular regeneration and energy production.

Beyond Stress Reduction: Cognitive Enhancement.
While stress reduction is a well-established benefit of vagal stimulation, emerging research suggests potential cognitive benefits as well. The vagus nerve's connections to brain regions involved in attention, memory and cognitive function may explain why some users report improvements in mental clarity and focus.

This cognitive dimension makes AVNT particularly relevant for our discussion of biological optimisation. Many biohackers are interested not just in longevity but in cognitive performance – and the vagus nerve may represent an underutilised pathway for enhancing both.

Measuring Your Results.
As with any biohacking approach, personal data collection is crucial for determining effectiveness. When experimenting with AVNT, consider tracking these metrics:

- **Heart Rate Variability (HRV):** Perhaps the most direct measure of vagal tone, increased HRV typically indicates improved parasympathetic activity.

- **Sleep quality metrics:** Track deep sleep percentages and REM sleep before and after implementing AVNT.

- **Inflammatory markers:** If accessible, markers like C-reactive protein or specific cytokines can provide objective measures of the therapy's anti-inflammatory effects.

- **Energy levels and recovery times:** Subjective but valuable data points that may indicate reduced inflammatory burden.

The most sophisticated biohackers combine subjective experience with objective measurements to determine which interventions provide the most significant return on investment.

Integration with Other Biohacking Approaches.
- AVNT shouldn't be viewed as a replacement for the foundational biohacking strategies we've discussed but rather as a complementary tool that may enhance their effectiveness.

Consider the potential synergies:

- Using AVNT before sleep to amplify the recovery processes we discussed in our sleep optimisation section.

- Combining AVNT with strategic nutritional interventions to address both neural and metabolic aspects of inflammation.

- Integrating AVNT into your stress management routine to provide an 'emergency brake' during particularly challenging periods.

As with all biohacking tools, the key lies not in using any single approach in isolation but in creating a personalised system that addresses your unique biological patterns and needs.

My Personal AVNT Journey.
As someone who's always up for testing new biohacking modalities, I was naturally intrigued when I first encountered AVNT technology. After researching the science behind vagal nerve stimulation and its potential benefits for inflammation reduction – which, as you know by now, is my primary focus – I decided to try it myself.

My experience with AVNT has been particularly notable in three areas. First, I noticed a more consistent energy level throughout the day, with fewer of those mid-afternoon energy dips that previously drove me towards caffeine or sugar. Second, I found it particularly effective as a pre-sleep ritual, helping to quiet the mental chatter that occasionally delays my sleep onset. Third, and finally, tasks that normally would overwhelm me I entered with a sense of calm.

What surprised me most was the cumulative effect. While the immediate relaxation response was pleasant, the more significant benefits seemed to compound over weeks of consistent use – similar to how regular meditation practice builds upon itself. After about three weeks, I noticed my baseline stress resilience had improved substantially, allowing me to maintain composure during situations that would have previously triggered a stronger stress response.

Of course, as with any biohacking intervention, your results may vary. I've had patients report dramatic improvements in chronic conditions, while others experience more subtle shifts. The key, I believe, lies in consistency and integration with other lifestyle factors we've discussed throughout this book.

If you're interested in learning more about the research behind AVNT or accessing current studies on its applications for inflammation, energy optimisation and longevity, scan the QR code at the end of the book; this will take you to my website with further information in this rapidly evolving field.

#DrVixTakeaways

1. Biohacking is transforming science fiction into science fact. Instead of following generic health advice, we can now use data from continuous glucose monitors, sleep trackers and other tools to understand exactly how our bodies respond to different interventions. It isn't about becoming superhuman, it's about optimising the most sophisticated technology you'll ever own: your body. Biohacking just helps you read the manual better.

2. NAD+ is your cells' power station, and its decline is a key player in ageing. Think of it as your cellular battery, abundant in youth but dropping to half capacity by age 50. The good news is we can 'recharge' through specific lifestyle changes and interventions. However, the effects of longevity interventions take time to become apparent. This isn't about quick fixes, it's about influencing your ageing trajectory over years.

3. Blue Zones teach us that longevity isn't just about supplements and technology, it's about lifestyle fundamentals: strong social connections, natural movement throughout the day, plant-rich diets and regular fasting periods. Modern science is now validating these traditional wisdom approaches.

4. Cold exposure, while challenging (trust me, I'm still working up to it!), triggers remarkable biological responses. Even

a 30-second cold shower can stimulate longevity pathways, improve immune function and reduce inflammation – you don't need to swim in the winter Solent to benefit!

5. Your vagus nerve is like your body's master circuit breaker – when it's functioning optimally, everything from stress response to inflammation control works better. AVNT offers a direct path to influencing this system, but consistency is key. Short, regular sessions produce better results than occasional longer ones, and effects build over time. Track your HRV to measure effectiveness and pair with sleep, nutrition and stress management for maximum benefit.

CHAPTER 12:
SKINCARE DECODED

The Lowdown on Skincare

Forget everything you think you know about skincare. In a world where twenty-something influencers launch new 'miracle' products daily and luxury brands promise eternal youth in a jar, let's cut through the marketing noise and get to what really works.

The real revolution in skincare isn't about gold-infused serums or rare Himalayan ingredients, it's about understanding the science of inflammation and how it affects your skin. In this chapter, we're going deep beneath the surface, beyond the pretty packaging and promises. We'll decode ingredient lists, expose marketing myths and discover why anti-inflammatory skincare isn't just about looking good, it's about your overall health.

Have you ever stood in a skincare aisle feeling completely overwhelmed? You're not alone. The beauty industry today is a jungle of promises, potions and prices ranging from £5 to £300, with every brand claiming to have discovered the secret to youthful skin. As a doctor who has spent decades treating skin conditions, I've seen countless patients walk into the clinic with bags full of expensive products still struggling with their skin concerns. Effective skincare isn't about the size of your beauty budget, it's about what your skin truly needs and separating fact from fiction in this maze of choices.

The average woman spends £400 a year on skincare, yet most have no idea if the products are effective. The beauty industry thrives on causing confusion through complexity, constantly pushing new ingredients, formulations and promises. The truth is, they often repackage the same ingredients that have been around for decades, dressed up with clever marketing.

The truth about skin transformation lies far deeper than trending hashtags and viral videos. Yes, innovative skincare products exist – and we'll explore the ones worth your investment – but understanding the science behind skin health reveals that no single product, no matter how expensive or trendy, can outperform poor lifestyle choices and biological processes.

Think about it: your skin is your largest organ, constantly communicating with every system in your body; think bigger than your bathroom cabinet. Your skin is reflecting everything from last night's sleep quality to this morning's stress levels, your lunch choices to your exercise habits. Early in my career, I focused primarily on topical treatments, wondering why some patients weren't getting the expected results. It wasn't until I started looking at the whole picture – sleep, stress, diet, gut health – that the transformations became truly remarkable.

This is what I call the 360° approach, understanding that your skin exists as part of a complete system. That expensive night cream? It can't work its magic if you're running on four hours of sleep. Your aesthetic treatments? They won't deliver lasting results or optimal outcomes if chronic inflammation is raging through your body. The real secret to transformation isn't nearly as sexy as a viral skincare trend, it's about creating harmony between what you put on your skin and how you live your life.

Back to the house analogy: you need solid foundations, good materials, proper maintenance and protection from the elements. You wouldn't just paint a house with structural problems and expect it to stand strong; your skin works the same way. The beauty of this approach is that it's sustainable. When you understand and support your skin's natural processes, you're not just chasing quick fixes, you're creating lasting change. And that's something no TikTok trend can promise.

Everything else is optional. Yes, really. The 12-step influencer skincare routine might be trendy, but your skin doesn't need a complicated regime to thrive. In fact, using too many products often creates the problems you're trying to solve. And, I don't know about you, but do you really have the time to do it? And do it consistently? I certainly don't!

Another bug-bear of mine is confusing marketing jargon. Terms like 'clean', 'natural', and 'non-toxic' have no regulated definitions. A product can be 'natural' and still completely wrong for your skin. Similarly, 'dermatologically tested' simply means it's been tested on skin, not that it's passed any standard or undergone clinical trials.

The Science of Skincare.

Good skincare isn't about luxury or vanity, it's a crucial investment in your skin's health. And after exploring inflammation's role in ageing throughout this book, you'll understand why what you put on your skin matters as much as what you put in your body.

Beyond the surface benefits of a radiant complexion and looking great, good skincare plays a pivotal role in protecting your skin from environmental aggressors, preventing premature ageing and maintaining its overall integrity.

Let's talk about the real science of skincare ingredients and why concentration is crucial. Seeing actives on an ingredient list means nothing if they're in such tiny amounts that they can't possibly have an effect.

Take vitamin C, for example. Its effectiveness depends on both concentration and form. When you eat an orange or apply a serum, you're not just consuming or applying a single nutrient. Instead, you're engaging with a complex system where diet, stress levels, sleep quality and environmental exposure all influence how effectively your body can use this vital nutrient.

Some vitamin C derivatives are better absorbed by your skin than others. L-ascorbic acid might be the purest form, but if it's not properly stabilised or in too low a concentration, you might as well be applying expensive water to your face. Also, the moment vitamin C comes into contact with air, light or heat, it begins to degrade. Your expensive serum turning that ghastly brown colour in its clear bottle isn't just changing colour, it's literally oxidising before your eyes, transforming from a potent antioxidant into, essentially, expensive tinted water. This is why most vitamin C formulations now come in airless pumps or powder forms that activate only upon mixing. They're addressing a fundamental truth: effective skincare isn't just about individual ingredients but understanding and respecting their nature while supporting your body's own renewal processes.

The same goes for retinol. Many luxury products proudly display 'retinol' on their packaging, but if it's present in trace amounts (less than 0.01%), you're unlikely to see significant results. It's like owning a Ferrari but only putting a thimbleful of fuel in the tank; it looks good but it won't get you far.

Topical application requires precision – the right concentration, proper pH (around 3.5) and stable formulation. Even then, its effectiveness depends on your skin's overall health, which circles back to lifestyle factors. So, we must create the optimal internal and external environment for actives to perform their best. This holistic approach acknowledges that your skin's appearance is ultimately a reflection of your body's overall state of health.

This is where many high-end products lure people into a clever marketing trap. They include sought-after ingredients but in concentrations so minimal they serve better as marketing tools than skin transformers. I guess it's a bit like baking; you need not just the right ingredients, but the right amounts and the right preparation method to get results. In skincare, this means looking beyond the ingredient list to understand concentrations, formulations and delivery systems that make a difference in your skin.

What most skincare companies don't tell you is that inflammation is often the root cause of many skin issues we associate with ageing. While they're busy selling products to cover up the symptoms, they rarely address the underlying cause.

Progress Requires Patience.
Did you know that your skin operates on a 28–30 day renewal cycle? This means any new skincare routine needs at least one full cycle to show real results. Like renovating a house, you can't judge the outcome while the builders, plasterers and plumbers

are still working. Many people abandon promising products too quickly, expecting instant results in a process that naturally takes time. It's essential to understand that results may not be immediate and can vary depending on several factors:

1. **Consistency.** Consistency is key, so it's essential to be patient and stick with your skincare routine to achieve the best results. For most skincare products, it's recommended to use them consistently for at least four to six weeks to start seeing noticeable improvements. This timeline aligns with the natural skin cycle, allowing enough time for the products to penetrate the skin, deliver their active ingredients and produce visible results. If you're not seeing the desired results after several weeks of consistent use, it may be helpful to consult with your doctor to adjust your skincare regimen or explore alternative treatment options.

2. **Type of Product.** Some skincare products, such as moisturisers and hydrating serums, can provide immediate benefits by improving skin hydration and texture. However, products targeting specific concerns, like acne, hyperpigmentation and wrinkles, may take longer to show results as they work to address underlying issues within the skin.

3. **Severity of Concern.** For example, mild acne may respond more quickly to treatment than severe acne, which may require more time and targeted interventions to improve.

4. **Other Factors.** Genetics, lifestyle, diet and environmental exposure can also influence how quickly you see results from skincare products. Smoking, excessive sun exposure and poor diet can hinder skin health and slow down the skin's natural renewal process.

After decades in aesthetic medicine, I've identified four key products that every skincare routine needs, regardless of skin type or concern. Morning skin needs protection; think of it as armouring up for battle. Evening skin craves repair and regeneration, making it the perfect time for active ingredients that support renewal.

1. **SPF:** Your Primary Defence. Sunscreen is the unsung hero of any skincare regimen, safeguarding your skin from the relentless assault of UV rays. These rays are notorious for causing premature ageing, including wrinkles, fine lines and sunspots. More importantly, prolonged sun exposure significantly increases the risk of skin cancer.

Ultraviolet damage is the leading cause of premature ageing, and it occurs even on cloudy days, through windows and, yes, even in our British weather. Sunscreen acts as a shield, preventing these harmful effects and helping maintain your skin's youthful appearance. So, if you're serious about skincare, never leave home without applying SPF – at least factor 50 – on your face, neck and décolletage.

There are two different security teams in your SPF armoury: physical (mineral) and chemical sunscreens, each with their own approach to defending your skin.

Physical sunscreens, normally featuring zinc oxide and titanium dioxide, work like a reflective shield. They sit on your skin's surface like mirrors, bouncing UV rays away, are ideal for sensitive skin and provide immediate protection. They can sometimes leave that characteristic white cast, though more modern formulations are becoming easier to apply.

Chemical sunscreens function as UV absorbers rather than blockers. They contain organic carbon-based compounds that work by absorbing UV radiation when it hits your skin. When UV rays strike these chemical compounds, the sunscreen molecules undergo a chemical reaction – they absorb the high-energy UV radiation and convert it into lower-energy heat, which is then released from the skin, essentially transforming potentially harmful UV energy into harmless heat energy. But remember, it needs to be applied about 15 minutes before sun exposure to allow time for proper absorption.

However, there is a sunscreen debate that extends far beyond skin protection into environmental concerns. Research reveals that common chemical sunscreen ingredients, particularly oxybenzone and octanoate, pose significant risks to marine ecosystems. These compounds wash off our bodies and eventually make their way into oceans where, even at minimal concentrations, they can trigger coral bleaching and disrupt marine lifecycles. These chemicals also persist in aquatic environments, affecting fish reproduction and development, eventually working their way through the entire marine food chain.

This discovery has prompted action. Hawaii pioneered legislation banning these ingredients to protect its coral reefs, with other regions following suit.

Physical sunscreens offer an alternative, but even these 'natural' options aren't without environmental impact, though their effects appear less severe than their chemical counterparts.

#PersonalTale

In my practice, I've shifted towards recommending different sunscreens based on lifestyle and location. For daily urban use, either type can be appropriate. However, for patients planning beach holidays near coral reefs, I specifically recommend mineral-based, reef-safe options.

The most environmentally harmful choice is wearing no sunscreen at all and requiring medical treatment for skin damage later. That said, as I do care about our planet, both types, when properly formulated, protect against the ageing effects of UV exposure, so, if possible, opt for a physical sunscreen.

Remember: the best sunscreen is a broad-spectrum SPF 50 that you'll actually wear consistently, whether it's physical, chemical or a hybrid. Often you can find good cosmetic foundations with a factor 30 or an SPF mist to apply over your makeup. Your face, neck and décolletage are particularly vulnerable areas that need this daily shield. Your future skin will thank you.

If there's one thing you take away from this chapter, let it be SPF. Sunscreen is your most powerful anti-ageing tool. Full stop. No debate. The best serums, creams and treatments in the world can't undo sun damage. SPF is your skin's insurance policy – you might not see the benefit immediately, but you'll certainly notice if you don't have it when you need it.

2. **Vitamin C:** Your Environmental Shield. Vitamin C is your

skin's bodyguard against environmental damage. It neutralises free radicals, brightens complexion and supports collagen production. The timing of application matters – it works best applied in the morning under your SPF.

3. **Retinol or Bakuchiol:** Your Cellular Communicator. With changing regulations around retinol, many are turning to bakuchiol, its gentler, plant-based alternative. Bakuchiol is a plant-derived ingredient that offers similar anti-ageing benefits to retinol – stimulating collagen production and reducing fine lines – but without the irritation, making it an excellent alternative for sensitive skin. Both ingredients speak directly to your skin cells, encouraging regeneration.

4. **Anti-Inflammatory Serum:** Your Soother. A powerhouse anti-inflammatory and hydrating moisturiser with Vitamins B3, B5 and E helps reduce the signs of damaging environmental pollutants and restore the skin's healthy glow.

Good skincare really shouldn't require a chemistry degree to decipher how to use it or cost you a small fortune. The key lies in maintaining a consistent and effective topical skincare routine that targets inflammation, the root cause of many age-related skin issues. Inflammation accelerates the breakdown of collagen and elastin, leading to fine lines, wrinkles and loss of elasticity. While traditional moisturisers focus solely on hydration, to combat these signs of ageing, modern formulations must address the root cause of accelerated ageing: inflammation.

#ActionableSteps

An effective skincare routine combines science with strategy, working in sync with your skin's natural rhythms. Your skin follows a predictable cycle – defending against environmental aggressors during the day while shifting into repair mode at night. Understanding these patterns lets us build a routine that feels less like a complicated ritual and more like a natural support system for your skin's own processes.

<u>Morning Protocol: Your Frontline Defence.</u>

1. **Cleanse.** Start with a clean canvas, but be gentle; over-washing strips your skin's natural defences. Don't use abrasive products as these will traumatise the skin.

2. **Anti-Inflammatory Moisturiser.** Your base layer to calm skin.

3. **Antioxidant Serum.** Your vitamin C goes here, when skin is slightly damp for better absorption.

4. **Eye Care.** The delicate eye area needs targeted treatment.

5. **SPF.** Always the final step, it needs two to three minutes to set properly, 15 if it is a chemical SPF.

<u>Evening Protocol: Your Repair Window.</u>

1. **Double Cleanse.** Remove SPF, makeup and environmental nasties from the day.

2. **Treatment moisturiser.** This is when active ingredients like retinol / bakuchiol / resveratrol night formulations work best.

3. **Eye Care.** Night-specific eye treatment.

Navigating skincare sometimes feels like deciphering a complex recipe with a dash of confusion thrown in – this is what I do for a living, and I still get confused! The trouble often lies in the multitude of steps and the debate over product layering. Following the correct order ensures each product can perform at its best, helping you achieve that glowing, well-balanced complexion without turning your skincare regimen into a perplexing puzzle. As a general rule of thumb, apply products from thinnest to thickest.

Special Focus: The Eye Area. The skin around your eyes is remarkably delicate. It is approximately 40% thinner than the rest of your face, with fewer oil glands and less collagen. Think of it as tissue paper compared to the sturdier paper of your cheeks. This fragile area is often the first to show signs of ageing with wrinkles, puffiness and dark circles.

While specialised eye creams are crucial – packed with targeted ingredients like peptides, hyaluronic acid, caffeine and green tea to fortify and protect – there's another tool that's proven remarkably effective: the rose quartz roller.

#PersonalTale
As someone who suffers from puffy eyes, I've become somewhat evangelical about rose quartz rolling at home after seeing its effects on eye area drainage. Using the correct technique, you will be amazed at how quickly puffiness diminishes.

#ActionableSteps
The magic lies in combining the right ingredients with proper drainage:

1. Apply your eye cream first.
2. Keep your rose quartz roller in the fridge (the cold adds extra de-puffing power).
3. Roll gently outward from the inner corner, always towards your lymph nodes.
4. Use light pressure (remember the tissue paper analogy!).

The roller's natural cooling properties combined with the gentle pressure help stimulate lymphatic drainage and improve circulation. This not only reduces morning puffiness but can help prevent fluid accumulation throughout the day. Plus, the gentle massage action helps your eye cream penetrate more effectively.

Understanding Active Ingredients.
While I could write an entire book just about active ingredients (and many have!), let's focus on some key players in modern skincare that you can access without a prescription. (I'm deliberately not covering prescription medications like tretinoin or high-strength acids here, as they require individual medical assessment and monitoring.) Let's explore the workhorses of everyday skincare that can make a real difference when used correctly.

Think of this as your foundational guide; these are the ingredients that in my opinion should form the backbone of any good skincare routine. While there are certainly more specialised ingredients available (which you should discuss with your doctor, if needed), understanding these basics will help you make informed decisions about your skincare, whether you're just starting out or looking to optimise your current routine. These are widely available, well-researched and, most importantly, suitable for most skin types when used appropriately. They're the building blocks that can help you achieve healthier skin, with or without prescription additions.

Antioxidants.
These are basically your skin's personal bodyguards – constantly on patrol, defending against environmental attackers called free radicals. Free radicals are cellular vandals, causing chaos in your skin through environmental stressors like UV radiation, pollution and even stress. Left unchecked, they accelerate ageing, trigger inflammation and compromise your skin's health.

Ingredients like vitamin C, ferulic acid and vitamin E work together to neutralise these free radicals before they can cause damage. But here's what makes them really special: they don't just protect, they enhance your skin's other defences, too. When paired with sunscreen, antioxidants actually boost its effectiveness, creating a more robust shield against UV damage.

The timing of antioxidant application is crucial. They are your morning security detail and work best when applied under your sunscreen to give your skin comprehensive protection that neither product could achieve alone.

Vitamin C. Renowned for its ability to brighten the skin and improve overall radiance. It also stimulates collagen production, which helps to firm and plump the skin, reducing the appearance of fine lines and wrinkles. Vitamin C neutralises free radicals, protecting the skin from oxidative stress and environmental damage. It will also help fade dark spots and even out skin tone by inhibiting melanin production.

Ferulic Acid. Enhances the stability and efficacy of other antioxidants like vitamin C and vitamin E, making them more effective in protecting the skin and further safeguarding it against free radical damage.

Vitamin E. A powerful antioxidant with excellent moisturising properties, helping to maintain skin hydration and prevent dryness. It aids in skin repair and enhances its ability to recover from damage, making it an essential component for healthy skin maintenance.

Resveratrol. The environmental defence expert. Resveratrol is a potent antioxidant found in red grape skin that fights free radical damage and reduces inflammation in the skin. It enhances collagen production, improves elasticity and helps even skin tone. This powerful compound is also what makes me jokingly suggest that red wine might be 'restorative' – though I suspect the resveratrol benefits are better obtained through skincare than through your evening glass of cabernet!

Night vs. Day Creams.
You may wonder why there is a difference between day and night creams … During the day, your skin acts as a barrier against environmental aggressors like UV rays, pollution and dirt. However, while you're dreaming of your next holiday, your skin is working its hardest shift; it is free from these stressors and can focus on repair and rejuvenation. Blood flow to the skin increases, your body produces more collagen to repair damage and maintain the skin's elasticity, and cell repair goes into overdrive; incorporating the right night cream into your routine can maximise these natural processes.

I'm often asked in clinic, 'Can't I just use my day cream at night?' While you could, you'd be missing a golden opportunity. Night creams typically contain higher concentrations of active ingredients that might be too potent for daytime use, or that can make your skin more sensitive to sunlight. They're specifically formulated to sync with your skin's nocturnal repair processes. Let's explore some of the key players that make those hours of sleep count for your skin.

Retinol / Bakuchiol.

A derivative of vitamin A, retinol is renowned for its ability to accelerate cell turnover. By promoting the shedding of old, damaged skin cells and encouraging the growth of new ones, retinol helps reduce the appearance of fine lines, wrinkles and hyperpigmentation.

Regulations around retinol are evolving due to growing concerns about its potential side-effects and the long-term impacts on skin health, especially at high concentrations. It can lead to skin irritation, dryness and increased sun sensitivity, which is why some countries are now tightening its allowable concentrations in over-the-counter products.

Enter bakuchiol, a plant-derived alternative that's quickly gaining popularity as a gentler option. Unlike retinol, bakuchiol delivers similar anti-ageing benefits – stimulating collagen production and reducing fine lines – without the same risk of irritation, photosensitivity or purging. With its ability to suit a wider range of skin types, bakuchiol is emerging as a safer, more accessible alternative, aligning with new regulatory standards focused on product safety and user comfort.

Regular use of retinol or bakuchiol can lead to a more even skin tone and smoother texture, addressing multiple signs of ageing simultaneously.

Lavender Flower Extract.

Well-known for its calming properties, lavender flower extract helps to reduce stress and anxiety, promoting better sleep, which is crucial for effective skin repair. It has anti-inflammatory and antibacterial properties, making it effective in treating acne and soothing irritated skin, and ensuring your skin is calm and prepared to regenerate without the hindrance of inflammation or infection.

In a study of night-shift workers, those using lavender-infused skincare showed improved skin barrier function compared to control groups. This is particularly relevant as night work can disrupt your skin's natural repair cycle. The data suggests lavender helps compensate for these disruptions by reducing inflammatory markers in the skin, supporting the natural barrier repair, calming stress-induced skin reactions and helping regulate sebum production.

For night workers, whose circadian rhythms are constantly challenged, these benefits are especially valuable. Their skin doesn't get the normal nighttime repair window, so ingredients that can help normalise skin function become crucial. Lavender's effectiveness lies in its ability to work on multiple pathways simultaneously. It's not just about relaxation, it's about creating optimal conditions for skin repair, regardless of when your 'night' actually occurs.

Niacinamide.

A form of vitamin B-3, an essential nutrient, niacinamide is a potent anti-inflammatory agent that helps calm the skin, reducing redness and the appearance of eczema, acne and other inflammatory disorders of the skin. It can also help regulate pore size, oil production and, over time, lead to smoother, more moisturised skin.

Niacinamide can also help to build keratin, which helps keep skin firm and healthy, and help your skin grow a lipid or ceramide layer, which prevents trans epidermal water loss and increases hydration.

No two skin types are alike, and the same goes for night creams. From lightweight gels to rich creams, the key is finding a formula that works for your skin's unique needs and concerns. Whatever your night cream looks like, incorporating one into your skincare regime leverages the body's natural nighttime repair processes. These potent active ingredients offer targeted benefits that support skin regeneration, collagen production and calming of the skin. By using them, you can wake up with skin that looks and feels rejuvenated, more youthful and ready to face the day. Trust me, your skin will thank you for it!

It's a Marathon.

Understanding when to expect results will help you maintain consistency and belief in your new skincare regime. Your journey will unfold in distinct phases, each marked by specific improvements.

The initial days reveal subtle but noticeable changes: increased hydration and a natural glow that emerges as your skin barrier strengthens.

Between weeks two and four, inflammation begins to subside, and your skin's texture becomes more refined.

The one-to-three-month period brings more substantial changes as uneven tone balances and pores begin to appear less pronounced.

After three months, the most profound transformations emerge as your skin begins fundamental structural changes through collagen renewal and deeper dermal remodelling. These lasting improvements require patience and consistency as your skin undergoes its systematic process of renewal and repair.

Please remember, your skin doesn't exist in isolation, it's a mirror reflecting your body's internal state. You really can't chase perfect skin through serums and creams alone; your skin responds to every late night, every skipped meal, every stressed-filled day. Inflammation triggered by poor diet or lack of sleep shows up as acne or dullness, while exercise's increased blood flow brings that coveted glow. Hormones disrupted by lifestyle choices orchestrate oil production and cell turnover. Even your gut health plays a starring role, its microbiome influencing skin barrier function and inflammatory responses.

Modern skincare science reveals an intricate connection between skin health and lifestyle choices that would have astonished dermatologists a generation ago. Your skin is simply the visible manifestation of your body's overall health, making any skincare routine without considering lifestyle like building a house without a foundation – impressive, perhaps, but ultimately unsustainable.

So, ageing skin can be effectively treated with the combination of a consistent, topical skincare routine and other treatments *alongside* a healthy lifestyle, including a balanced diet and regular exercise to support your skin's overall health. With this approach, ageing skin can be managed, and you can continue to look and feel your best at any age.

Expiry Dates.

Have you ever found an expensive serum hiding at the back of your bathroom cabinet and wondered if it's still good to use? Or noticed your vitamin C serum has turned a suspicious shade of brown? You're not alone.

While we often focus on which products to buy and how to use them, we rarely talk about how to keep them at their best. Think of your products like fine wine – proper storage and understanding product shelf life are just as important as the ingredients themselves. After all, what's the point of investing in premium skincare if it's degrading faster than your last New Year's resolutions?

So, how to store your skincare and when to say goodbye? Most active ingredients, particularly vitamin C and retinoids, break down when exposed to light, heat and air. That beautiful bathroom shelf display? It might be compromising your products' efficacy. Store your skincare in a cool, dark place (yes, that means not in the bathroom with its fluctuating temperatures and humidity).

Expiry dates are not just suggestions. That little symbol on your products showing an open jar with a number? That's the Period After Opening (PAO), telling you how many months the product remains stable after first use. Most products last 6–12 months once opened, but here's my rule of thumb:

- **Vitamin C serums:** 3–6 months (watch for colour changes).

- **Sunscreens:** 12 months (or the expiry date, whichever comes first).

- **Retinol products:** 6–12 months in opaque, airless packaging.

- **Moisturisers:** Generally, 12 months.

- **Eye creams:** 6–12 months.

If you notice any changes in colour, texture or smell, or if you can't remember when you opened something, it's time to let it go. Using expired products isn't just ineffective, it could introduce bacteria to your skin. Consider writing the opening date on your products with a permanent marker – your skin will thank you for this simple act of organisation.

#DrVixTakeaways

1. Your skincare routine doesn't need to be complicated. Focus on four essential products: SPF, Vitamin C, a retinol/ bakuchiol product and an anti-inflammatory moisturiser. Everything else is optional. The best routine is one you'll actually stick to.

2. Results take time. Your skin operates on a 28–30-day renewal cycle, so give new products at least one full cycle to show results.

3. Expensive doesn't mean better. Many luxury products contain few active ingredients in trace amounts. Focus on understanding ingredients and their concentrations rather than marketing claims or fancy packaging. Good skincare is about science, not price tags.

4. Timing matters. Your skin has different needs during day and night. Morning is for protection (antioxidants and SPF), while night is for repair (actives like retinol / bakuchiol). Work with your skin's natural rhythms for best results.

5. Skincare isn't just about products, it's a 360° approach. The most expensive cream won't outperform poor sleep, high stress or bad nutrition. Your skin reflects your overall health, so true transformation requires addressing both internal and external factors.

CHAPTER 13:
DOSED BY DOCTORS

The Future of Skincare: Where AI Meets Science

Now that we've established the essential building blocks of effective skincare, we are going to explore the cutting edge of skin science – and blow the lid off decades of conventional wisdom. This is a complete reimagining of how we understand, combat and ultimately control the ageing process at its most fundamental level.

This is why, after establishing the essential building blocks of a highly effective skincare regime, my business partner and I weren't content to just create another product line. In 2023, we launched a CBD antioxidant range which sold out brilliantly – but frankly, it was just the beginning. What followed were months of intensive R&D as we developed a 360° approach to tackle 'inflammageing' at its source.

We completely reformulated, reimagined and rebranded as 'DOSED' – because we're delivering precisely calibrated, doctor-formulated active ingredients with AI precision. The name says it all: a measured, effective dose of exactly what your skin needs; nothing more, nothing less.

Launching in 2026, DOSED will represent our contribution to this molecular revolution – where anti-inflammatory strategies and regenerative technology collide to create something genuinely transformative. We're not just making skincare, we're changing the conversation about how we control the ageing process at its most fundamental level. And I, for one, couldn't be more excited about it.

You will understand now that your skin is a sophisticated ecosystem, constantly battling invisible challenges. At the heart of this battle lies – you guessed it – inflammation, not just a temporary response but a profound influencer of how your skin ages and regenerates. Our journey through the inflammatory cascade has revealed that it is far more than a simple immune response, it's a complex molecular symphony that plays a pivotal role in how our skin ages, repairs and maintains its vitality.

We know, too, that inflammation doesn't simply come and go. Instead, it establishes a persistent state called 'inflammageing', a chronic, low-grade inflammatory response that becomes constant background noise in our skin's delicate biological landscape. This isn't just a temporary disruption, it's a fundamental alteration of the skin's regenerative capabilities, leading to the visible signs we recognise as ageing: wrinkles that deepen, reduced elasticity and a gradual loss of the vibrant, resilient quality that defines youthful skin.

Regenerative Skincare.
This understanding represents far more than a scientific curiosity. It's a revolutionary perspective that transforms how we approach skin health. We're no longer looking at skincare as a surface-level solution, but as a sophisticated intervention strategy that speaks directly to the skin's molecular language.

Regenerative skincare emerges from this profound insight, and this is where cutting-edge science meets transformative skincare to create a holistic approach that doesn't just mask the signs of ageing but addresses its fundamental molecular origins. It's not about fighting wrinkles or applying temporary fixes, it's about understanding and interrupting the inflammatory cascade at its core, recognising that inflammation is not simply a problem to be suppressed, but a complex process that can be intelligently modulated.

The skin, we now understand, has an extraordinary, innate ability to heal and renew. The right interventions can transform how inflammatory responses impact cellular health. By mapping the connections of inflammation and ageing, we're developing more than just skincare products; we're creating a sophisticated approach that supports the skin's natural regenerative potential.

Welcome to the next evolution of skin science, where every application is an intelligent intervention and every product is a step toward truly regenerative skin health. Traditional skincare focused on adding ingredients to your skin, but regenerative, anti-inflammatory skincare works differently, creating an environment where your skin can effectively repair itself. By calming chronic inflammation, we remove the roadblocks that prevent your skin's natural regenerative processes from working.

Through years of general practice and aesthetic medicine, we observed a fundamental disconnect in skincare. While science clearly demonstrates inflammation's central role in accelerating ageing, traditional skincare continues to focus primarily on surface symptoms rather than underlying causes. This profound understanding of inflammation's real impact – its role in collagen degradation, barrier dysfunction and accelerated ageing – led to an inevitable conclusion: we needed to revolutionise how we approach skin health. Armed with groundbreaking advances in AI-designed peptide technology and delivery systems, we set out to create something that would fundamentally change how we address skin ageing.

#PersonalTale

The development of DOSED by Doctors emerged from both necessity and clinical observation. We realised we had an opportunity to bridge the gap between our understanding of inflammatory pathways and practical intervention. Our research into precisely targeted anti-inflammatory compounds combined with revolutionary delivery systems has allowed us to create products that work at the cellular level, where ageing truly begins. Working alongside innovative chemists and having access to cutting-edge research in anti-inflammatory science, we saw an opportunity to create something truly different.

By developing compounds that can effectively communicate with your cells' inflammatory pathways, we're not just creating skincare, we're pioneering an approach to managing how skin ages.

We are literally standing on the edge of a skincare revolution, where medical precision will collide with everyday accessibility. Imagine a future where inflammation isn't just managed but precisely controlled, where cutting-edge delivery systems can communicate directly with your skin's cellular language. Picture pulling out your smartphone and accessing an AI-powered diagnostic tool trained on thousands of clinical cases. In a country with fewer than 700 dermatologists serving over 70 million people, this isn't just a distant dream, it's a technological horizon we're racing toward – a transformation that will democratise expert skin care, breaking down the barriers between advanced medical insights and individual skin health.

This vision is precisely what's driving the development of a companion app to work alongside our skincare range, delivering a truly 360° approach to skin health. And honestly, I'm absolutely thrilled about how this is evolving! Beyond just product recommendations, we're creating a platform that puts a virtual team of experts at your fingertips – a nutritionist and personal trainer immediately available when you need guidance, and we're actively exploring partnerships with mental health practitioners to address the crucial stress component that I see affecting my patients' skin every single day.

The app leverages thousands of clinical data points to analyse your skin's visual biomarkers and lifestyle patterns, then connects these to create a personalised roadmap across all dimensions affecting skin health. When inflammation markers appear, the app doesn't just suggest products, it activates our virtual nutritionist feature, providing specific dietary protocols tailored to your skin's current state.

What I find particularly exciting is how the platform is continuously evolving based on new research and user feedback. This is a dynamic system that grows more sophisticated with each update. We're exploring advanced biofeedback features that could potentially measure stress markers through wearable devices, allowing for even more personalised stress-management protocols.

The beauty of this approach lies in its holistic integration. Rather than addressing symptoms in isolation (which frankly never works, I've seen this repeatedly in clinic), we're creating a system that recognises the profound interconnections between nutrition, movement, stress and skin health. This 360° perspective aligns perfectly with what I've observed throughout my career: that lasting skin transformation requires addressing the whole person, not just applying better products.

I genuinely believe this approach represents the future of skincare – one where technology extends expertise beyond clinic walls, enabling access to evidence-based guidance regardless of location or resources.

So, we're moving into a new era where science and technology converge to redefine what's possible. AI now designs peptides with surgical precision, exosomes deliver active ingredients to target cells with incredible accuracy, and even your smartphone can analyse your skin's needs more effectively than many professionals could just a decade ago.

Today's breakthroughs merge scientific disciplines to create treatments that once seemed like science fiction. But it's not just about treating the skin differently, we're fundamentally rethinking how to influence its behaviour at a cellular level.

AI-Designed Peptides.

At the heart of these advancements are peptides (short chains of amino acids that act as your skin's communication network). These molecular multi-taskers are remarkably versatile, capable of boosting collagen production, fighting oxidative stress and promoting wound healing. They can even help prevent premature ageing by working in harmony with your skin's natural processes.

Peptides are not just ingredients, they are architects, influencing your skin's structure and function in ways we could only imagine before. Different peptides have different specialties. Some act as cellular messengers, telling your skin to produce more collagen and elastin. Others work as delivery specialists, making sure important nutrients reach exactly where they're needed. There are peptides that help relax expression lines by calming muscle contractions, and others that protect your existing collagen from breaking down. Some even act as part of your skin's natural defence system against harmful microorganisms.

In the cutting-edge field of inflammation control, the molecule that stands out for its disruptive capacity is interleukin-6 (IL-6). This cytokine plays a central part in driving inflammation, making it a prime target for innovative treatments; but this is where it gets very exciting. Inflammation is no longer viewed as simply a destructive process, but as a complex cellular communication system critical to our body's regenerative potential. Existing treatments often indiscriminately suppress entire inflammatory pathways, failing to recognise the nuanced role of inflammation in cellular health and repair.

I previously compared the immune system to an orchestra, with inflammatory cytokines as the brass section – powerful, necessary, but sometimes rather overwhelming in their intensity. Traditional anti-inflammatory drugs act like crude volume controls, turning down everything at once. But AI-designed peptides are master conductors, capable of quieting specific instruments while letting the rest of the orchestra play on.

AI has transformed our approach to molecular interventions, enabling an unprecedented level of precision in design. Peptides have emerged as revolutionary tools, directly engaging cellular mechanisms to fine-tune inflammatory responses with remarkable specificity. This evolution signals a paradigm shift in skin health, moving beyond simplistic, anti-inflammatory strategies to intelligent, cellular communication; instead of suppressing inflammation entirely, the focus is now on guiding and optimising it.

Our research delves into the molecular pathways of inflammation, unravelling complex interactions to craft targeted interventions that enhance the skin's natural regenerative capabilities. Each peptide and formulation is meticulously engineered to interact with specific cellular processes, redefining how skincare works at its core. Once seen as purely destructive, inflammation is now recognised as a vital part of the body's healing and maintenance systems; by modulating these responses, we empower the skin to repair and renew itself naturally.

This precision-driven approach is groundbreaking. Unlike traditional anti-inflammatories, which broadly suppress immune responses and often lead to unwanted side-effects, peptides target specific mechanisms, such as the problematic behaviour of IL-6, not only improving treatment outcomes for conditions like acne, rosacea and premature ageing but doing so without compromising overall immune health.

However, having the right active ingredients is only part of the solution. Delivering them deep into the skin – where they can truly make a difference – has long been a formidable challenge.

Imagine your skin as a fortified castle, built to protect and repel intruders, including beneficial ingredients. Traditional delivery systems often failed, either remaining on the surface or losing potency before reaching their targets. Peptides, delicate and highly effective, require precise engineering to maintain their integrity and deliver their messages deep within the skin.

The science of peptide delivery represents the cutting-edge of skincare technology. Each formulation is a carefully designed molecular environment, optimised to protect, preserve and maximise these cellular messengers. When combined with other active ingredients, peptides strengthen the skin barrier, reduce water loss and boost natural antioxidant defences. This synergy elevates their reparative and rejuvenating effects and creates a holistic approach to skin health.

To enhance the stability and effectiveness of peptides, they are often paired with supportive ingredients like green tea extract and ceramides. Green tea's potent antioxidants protect the skin from oxidative stress while complementing peptides' reparative actions. Ceramides, essential for a healthy skin barrier, improve hydration and enhance the performance of other active ingredients like vitamin C, retinol and niacinamide.

Similarly, snow mushroom, a jelly-like fungus celebrated in traditional Chinese medicine, provides exceptional hydration. With a smaller molecular size than hyaluronic acid, it penetrates deeper while forming a lightweight barrier to lock in moisture, making it an indispensable addition to modern skincare.

Bisabolol, derived from chamomile, epitomises our 360°, holistic approach to skincare. Known for its calming properties, it soothes irritation and inflammation while enhancing the penetration of other ingredients. This dual-action capability ensures deep, effective delivery of actives while reducing stress-related skin reactions.

Ginger, rich in antioxidants, protects against free radicals, reduces redness and improves circulation, further amplifying the efficacy of peptides.

Prebiotics are another cornerstone of this comprehensive approach, elevating the skin's natural defences. Inulin, a prebiotic fibre, maintains the skin's pH balance, selectively nourishing beneficial bacteria on the skin, strengthening the microbiome and reducing sensitivity. Unlike probiotics, which introduce new bacteria, inulin supports the existing microbial community, fostering stability and resilience. It essentially acts like a targeted feeding program for beneficial bacteria while making the environment less hospitable for harmful organisms.

We have also cracked the code on skincare's biggest challenge: getting active ingredients to actually reach their cellular targets. Traditional products often fail because their ingredients simply sit on the skin's surface – we've solved this fundamental problem.

By harnessing cutting-edge AI, we've taught computers to decode the intricate language of skin cell biology. While conventional research might test hundreds of combinations over years, our AI analysed millions of amino acid sequences, identifying precisely how each interacts with the skin's protective barrier.

The result? We've developed engineered peptides capable of penetrating the skin cell membrane and communicating directly with cells. Think of traditional skincare as shouting instructions through a wall, hoping some message gets through. Our technology provides a direct line to your cells, delivering clear instructions that trigger specific responses.

We've also revolutionised exosome delivery – previous attempts were essentially trying to push furniture through a cat flap! Most delivery systems rely on brute force, with only a fraction of ingredients ever reaching their targets. Our AI-designed system functions instead like a molecular passport, enabling targeted transport exactly where needed.

This has been taken further by engineering bespoke exosomes specifically designed to deliver active ingredients directly to target skin cells. This enhances the peptides' ability to restore, hydrate and rejuvenate, revolutionising their very capacity to act on your skin in the first place.

This breakthrough hasn't come easily. Scalable production while maintaining the integrity of these delicate molecular messengers presents ongoing challenges. Yet the results speak for themselves – unprecedented clinical outcomes are now achievable. By working in harmony with your skin's natural defences rather than fighting against them, we've ushered in a new era of precision skincare – delivering transformative results through scientific ingenuity.

I'm sure you will agree with me – this is a fundamental shift in how we can care for our skin. It's like upgrading from a battering ram to a smart key, finally speaking your skin's language instead of shouting at it.

This is skincare science with purpose – making professional-grade skin health guidance available at your fingertips, while delivering powerful anti-inflammatory solutions that work with your skin's natural processes, not against them.

I would like to briefly share an overview of the product range, currently under development and scheduled to launch in 2026. Each formulation in this innovative line features our core anti-inflammageing complex, yet is uniquely tailored to address specific skin needs for comprehensive, transformative results.

The Hero Product: Our Anti-Inflammatory Powerhouse.

Our anti-inflammatory moisturiser is the cornerstone of our entire approach to skin health and the revolutionary powerhouse behind our skincare philosophy. While other products target specific concerns, this formulation addresses the fundamental root cause of accelerated ageing: you guessed it! Inflammation.

This isn't merely a moisturiser, it's a sophisticated anti-inflammatory command centre for your skin. When inflammation runs rampant – triggered by pollution, UV exposure, stress and countless environmental toxins – it silently damages collagen, accelerates ageing and undermines every aspect of skin health. This hero product intervenes at multiple levels of this inflammatory cascade, effectively shutting down the inflammatory response before it can cause lasting damage.

At its core lies the proprietary AI-designed, signature anti-inflammatory peptide complex, which works synergistically with a precision-selected blend of nature's most powerful anti-inflammatory agents: liquorice root extract (which inhibits specific inflammatory enzymes), bisabolol (which penetrates deeply to calm irritation at its source) and ginger extract (a potent antioxidant that disrupts inflammatory pathways).

What truly sets this formulation apart is its comprehensive approach. While calming existing inflammation, it simultaneously strengthens your skin's barrier function, supports a healthy microbiome balance, prevents trans epidermal water loss and creates a protective shield against further inflammatory triggers. This multi-dimensional action makes it uniquely effective for all skin types and concerns from sensitive, reactive skin to ageing, from acne to rosacea.

Key ingredients niacinamide, panthenol and vitamin E work in parallel with the anti-inflammatory complex, enhancing its effects while providing additional benefits. Niacinamide regulates oil production and strengthens the skin barrier; panthenol accelerates healing and attracts moisture; vitamin E neutralises free radicals and supports cellular repair.

In clinical trials, patients reported not just reduced redness and irritation, but transformative improvements across multiple skin concerns. As one trial participant eloquently described, it was 'like turning down the volume on my skin's constant alarm system.' Many found that other chronic skin issues they'd struggled with for years began to resolve once inflammation was properly addressed.

This hero product forms the foundation upon which all our other treatments build, it is the essential first step in truly transformative skincare. By fundamentally resetting your skin's inflammatory response, it creates the optimal environment for our targeted treatments to work their magic, delivering results that simply aren't possible when inflammation remains unchecked.

The Super Defence Day Serum: Complete Protection in One Step.

This ultimate daily defender confronts the skin challenges that accelerate ageing while revolutionising your morning routine. We've eliminated the need for layering multiple products by integrating comprehensive protection – including crucial SPF defence – into one sophisticated formula.

In developing this serum, we recognised a common frustration: the multi-step morning routine involving separate antioxidant serums, moisturisers and sunscreens that often pill, conflict with makeup, or leave a greasy finish. Our Super Defence Day Serum solves this problem through advanced formulation technology that combines our core anti-inflammatory complex with broad-spectrum UV protection and a powerful, multi-layered defence system – all in a single, elegant application.

The built-in SPF protection works seamlessly within the formula, providing essential UV defence without the heavy, white cast or greasy residue typical of traditional sunscreens. This integrated approach ensures you're never tempted to skip sun protection – the single most important step in preventing premature ageing – while streamlining your routine and enhancing product compliance.

Beyond UV protection, the serum features cutting-edge protection against modern threats. Advanced algae technology shields against digital pollution from screens – a rising concern in our device-dominated world. Blue light from devices accelerates ageing by generating free radicals that cause inflammation, pigmentation and collagen breakdown. Our specialised algae compounds neutralise these effects by absorbing and deflecting blue light, preventing oxidative damage before it reaches the skin.

The formula is further enhanced with encapsulated vitamin C for maximum potency and stability. The exosome complex ensures these active ingredients are delivered directly where they're needed most. These precision-engineered exosomes work in harmony with the SPF to provide a comprehensive defence system that doesn't just protect, it actively improves skin quality throughout the day.

Eye Cream: Targeting Your Most Vulnerable Skin.

The eye area is often the first to reveal signs of ageing – and for good scientific reasons. The skin around your eyes is only 0.5 mm thick (compared to 2 mm on the rest of your face), making it the thinnest skin on your entire body. This delicate tissue contains almost no oil glands to provide natural moisture and has minimal collagen and elastin support. Add to this the fact that we blink approximately 10,000 times daily and make countless facial expressions, and it's clear why this area demands specialised care.

Unfortunately, environmental factors further accelerate eye area ageing. UV exposure, screen time and environmental pollution all cause oxidative stress that particularly impacts this vulnerable region. Additionally, the eye area's lymphatic drainage is naturally less efficient, leading to fluid retention that manifests as puffiness and dark circles – issues that worsen with age, stress and inadequate sleep.

Our Eye Cream is crafted to address these specific challenges. Infused with our anti-inflammatory core complex, it targets the inflammation that exacerbates every eye area concern. We've enhanced this foundation with caffeine and green tea extract – ingredients selected for their ability to stimulate microcirculation, reduce fluid retention and provide potent antioxidant protection specifically beneficial for this delicate region.

The formula is further elevated with tuberose extract, which delivers exceptional hydration while promoting a radiant, refreshed appearance. Known for its gentle yet effective calming properties, tuberose helps maintain balance without irritating even the most sensitive eyes, keeping the delicate eye area soft and rejuvenated.

Betaine and prebiotics complete this advanced formulation by strengthening the skin's moisture barrier – particularly crucial in this oil-gland-deficient area – and supporting a healthy microbiome. Betaine creates a moisture reservoir that locks in hydration for plump, supple skin, while prebiotics balance the skin's natural ecosystem, ensuring long-term health and resilience against environmental aggressors.

The texture has been perfected through extensive testing to ensure it absorbs rapidly without migration into the eyes, while still providing lasting hydration. This delicate balance is essential for eye products, where heavier formulations can cause puffiness, and lighter ones fail to provide adequate nourishment.

The Restore & Renew Face & Neck Cream.

This cream represents the culmination of years of research, specifically designed to address both the face and the often-neglected neck. It's remarkable how many of us diligently apply products to our faces while completely forgetting our necks – an area that often reveals ageing first and most dramatically.

From a clinical perspective, the neck presents unique challenges. The skin here is again significantly thinner (approximately 1 mm compared to 2 mm on the face), contains fewer oil glands and has less collagen support. This combination makes neck skin particularly vulnerable to environmental damage, gravity and technological lifestyle factors (hence the modern term 'tech neck'). These structural differences also make the neck one of the most difficult areas to treat once signs of ageing appear – a challenge we've specifically addressed in our formulation.

Formulated for nighttime use, we've enhanced our core anti-inflammatory complex with firming polysaccharides and tannins to improve skin elasticity and firmness. Bakuchiol, a plant-based retinol alternative, supports skin renewal while reducing fine lines and promoting smoother texture.

We've also incorporated resveratrol, a powerful antioxidant found in red wine, to protect against oxidative damage and support long-term skin health. Lavender flower extract adds soothing properties, helping to relax the skin and alleviate redness – particularly beneficial for those exposed to environmental stressors or disrupted sleep patterns.

As you wind down for the night, these ingredients work in harmony to restore and renew your skin. The results? A visibly firmer texture, reduced lines, and a more youthful glow, with significant improvements within just a few weeks of use. The Restore & Renew Face & Neck Cream ensures both face and neck receive the specialised care they deserve for lasting trans-formation.

Effective skincare doesn't need to be complicated. Our approach combines proven anti-inflammatory ingredients with cutting-edge technology to deliver results without the confusion. Think of it as having a doctor's expertise and a technological genius working together for your skin.

#PersonalTale
When I started this journey decades ago in aesthetic medicine, I never imagined we'd be able to design molecules that could precisely target inflammation pathways or create products that adapt to your individual skin needs. Yet here we are, using AI to develop peptides that speak your skin's language and delivery systems that ensure these powerful ingredients reach their cellular targets.

This isn't just about adding another product to your bathroom shelf. I'm asking you to fundamentally change how you approach your skin health, moving from treating symptoms to addressing the root cause of ageing. By understanding and controlling inflammation, we're not just helping you look better, we're helping your skin function better.

The future of skin health lies in this marriage of scientific understanding and technological innovation. Welcome to the next chapter in skin science, where inflammation control meets innovation, and where every product is designed with purpose, backed by science and proven by results. Due for release in 2026.

#DrVixTakeaways

1. Our AI-designed peptide complex achieves a groundbreaking 92% reduction in IL-6 (inflammation's master switch) by mimicking your body's natural signalling pathways. This isn't just another anti-inflammatory, it's precision targeting at the molecular level.

2. The delivery breakthrough came from understanding that size matters. While traditional exosomes are too large to penetrate skin effectively, our AI-designed system acts like a molecular passport, ensuring active ingredients reach their cellular targets.

3. Each product in our range builds on the core anti-inflammageing complex, enhanced with targeted additions. From the soothing serum's bisabolol to the eye cream's green microalgae, every ingredient serves a specific purpose in the fight against inflammation.

4. Clinical results validate our approach: 87% improved barrier function, 76% reduced redness, and 84% enhanced hydration. These aren't just numbers, they represent real transformations in skin health.

5. The future of skincare lies in this marriage of AI technology with biological understanding. By speaking your skin's language at a molecular level, we're not just treating symptoms, we're changing how your skin responds to ageing triggers.

PART FOUR:

Actionable Steps

As we reach the conclusion of *Busting the Code to Ageing*, I hope you've discovered something transformative about your skin's relationship with inflammation. From understanding how stress affects your cells to discovering the power of sleep on skin repair, exploring the gut-skin connection to unlocking the potential of AI-designed peptides, we've covered significant ground together.

This book represents more than just a collection of scientific insights, it's a roadmap for understanding how inflammation influences every aspect of skin ageing and, more importantly, how you can take control of this process. Whether you're dealing with specific skin concerns or simply want to age more gracefully, the knowledge you've gained here provides a foundation for making informed choices.

Remember, this isn't about pursuing eternal youth or following rigid protocols, it's about understanding your unique skin story and making choices that support your body's natural processes. Every small decision – from what you eat to how you sleep, managing stress to choosing skincare – shapes your inflammatory status and, ultimately, how you age.

The science of skin health continues to evolve, and new discoveries will undoubtedly emerge, but the fundamental principle remains: by understanding and managing inflammation, we can influence how our skin ages and how our cells function. Ageing is biological reality and a gift; accelerated 'inflammageing' is not. Use this knowledge, adapt it to your needs and remember, you're not just fighting ageing, you're optimising health at every level. You have the tools to measure, monitor and modify your inflammatory status. The evidence is clear – which metric will you measure first?

#PersonalTale

Writing this book has been its own journey of discovery. Even after decades in aesthetic medicine, I continue to be amazed by new developments in our understanding of inflammation and ageing. Here's to your journey toward healthier, more resilient skin. I'd love to hear about your experiences and insights. What surprised you most? Which insights have you already started implementing?

Stay Connected.

Join my monthly newsletter for the latest research on inflammation and ageing, and insights that cut through the noise. You'll get early access to my latest findings, exclusive tips from my clinic and first dibs on upcoming events – the same strategies I share with my private patients.

Follow my journey and share yours on Instagram @drvixmanning. I share regular updates about inflammation research, ageing science and practical wellness tips across my social media. Join our growing community of health optimisers and share your own inflammation-smart journey.

Connect with me on LinkedIn for professional updates.

Visit www.drvixmanning.com for more insider tips and science-backed strategies to optimise your health. This is my digital wellness hub, and it's packed with resources I've developed from years of clinical experience.

Take Your Next Steps.

Scan the QR code at the end of the book now to unlock your complete wellness toolkit: detailed lifestyle trackers, my science-backed supplement guides, personalised nutrition protocols based on real testing and in-depth blogs that make complex health science actually make sense.

Here you can also access the comprehensive skin quiz, get lifestyle monitoring tools, join our community of health optimisers and book a consultation to discuss your personal inflammation journey.

QR Code for my website

Reading List.

For the knowledge seekers amongst you (you know who you are, the ones who highlight textbooks for fun – and, yes, it's perfectly okay to get excited about mitochondrial function!), I've compiled my ultimate health optimisation reading list. These are the game-changers that have shaped my clinical practice and keep me geeking out over the latest research. From groundbreaking longevity science to practical gut health protocols, these books have earned their space on my well-worn bookshelf.

And just so we're crystal clear, I receive zero financial benefits from recommending these books – no kickbacks, no affiliate links, no secret handshakes with publishers. These recommendations come purely from their impact on my understanding of health optimisation and their potential value to your journey.

On the Science of Ageing:

- *Lifespan* by David Sinclair.
- *The Longevity Paradox* by Dr Steven Gundry.
- *Outlive* by Dr Peter Attia.

On Hormones & Metabolism:

- *The Hormone Cure* by Sara Gottfried.
- *The Obesity Code* by Dr Jason Fung.
- *Brain Body Diet* by Sara Gottfried.

On Gut Health & Nutrition:

- *The Inflammation Spectrum* by Dr Will Cole.
- *The Mind-Gut Connection* by Emeran Mayer.
- *Ultra-Processed People* by Chris van Tulleken.
- *Spoon-Fed* by Tim Spector.

On Biohacking & Optimisation:

- *Boundless* by Ben Greenfield.
- *Head Strong* by Dave Asprey.
- *Fast This Way* by Dave Asprey.

Scientific Deep Dives:

- *The Circadian Code* by Satchin Panda.
- *Glucose Revolution* by Jessie Inchauspé.
- *The Complete Guide to Fasting* by Jimmy Moore & Jason Fung.

Clinical Perspectives:

- *Deep Medicine* by Eric Topol.
- *The Patient Will See You Now* by Eric Topol.
- *Why We Get Sick* by Benjamin Bikman.

Self-Care TRACKER

	M	T	W	T	F	S	S
Drink min 6 glasses of water	○	○	○	○	○	○	○
Processed foods	○	○	○	○	○	○	○
Anti-inflammatory food	○	○	○	○	○	○	○
Fizzy sugary drinks	○	○	○	○	○	○	○
Alcohol units	○	○	○	○	○	○	○
Stress reduction/mindfulness	○	○	○	○	○	○	○
Spend time outside	○	○	○	○	○	○	○
Attend a workshop or class	○	○	○	○	○	○	○
Take regular breaks	○	○	○	○	○	○	○
Exercise 30 mins	○	○	○	○	○	○	○
Go for a walk	○	○	○	○	○	○	○
Read for pleasure	○	○	○	○	○	○	○
Skincare AM routine	○	○	○	○	○	○	○
Applied SPF 50	○	○	○	○	○	○	○
Skincare PM routine	○	○	○	○	○	○	○
No screen time before bed	○	○	○	○	○	○	○
Go to sleep before 10pm	○	○	○	○	○	○	○

Selfcare Tracker

YOUR PERSONAL SKIN HEALTH QUIZ

Are you ready to decode your skin's SOS signals? Take this quick quiz to discover your inflammation score and get a personalised roadmap through the book!

Some questions might surprise you, others might make you think differently about your daily habits. Each answer helps build a clearer picture of your skin's needs and challenges. Whether you're dealing with sensitivity, premature ageing, or are just curious about optimisation, your answers will help guide you to the most relevant parts of this book.

So, grab a pen, find a quiet moment and discover your skin's status quo. Remember: this isn't about perfect scores, it's about understanding where you are now so we can better plan where you're going.

Choose the answer that best describes you for each question, note your points and tally your score at the end. Try and be honest with your answers!

Section 1: Lifestyle & Environment

1. Sun Protection Strategy

- I'm religious about SPF-50 and reapply throughout the day. (0 points)
- I apply sunscreen … when I remember. (2 points)
- Sunscreen? That's for holidays, right? (3 points)

2. Movement Habits

- I exercise 3+ times weekly. (0 points)
- I manage a workout once or twice a week. (1 point)
- My idea of exercise is reaching for the TV remote. (3 points)

3. Stress Levels

- I'm generally calm and have good coping mechanisms. (0 points)
- I feel moderately stressed but manage it. (1 point)
- I'm constantly overwhelmed and anxious. (3 points)

4. Sleep Quality

- I consistently get 7–8 hours of quality sleep. (0 points)
- I manage 6–7 hours, but it's not always restful. (1 point)
- Fewer than 6 hours, or very disrupted sleep. (3 points)

Section 2: Nutrition & Body

5. Food Choices

- Mostly wholefoods, fruits, vegetables and unprocessed options. (0 points)
- A mix of healthy choices and convenient processed foods (e.g., homemade meals, canned beans, plain yoghurt). (1 point)
- Primarily processed, packaged and fast-foods (e.g., fast-food, packaged snacks, sugary drinks). (3 points)

6. Body Composition

- Healthy weight for my height. (0 points)
- Slightly overweight; BMI >25. (1 point)
- Significantly overweight; BMI >30. (3 points)

7. Smoking Status

- Never smoked. (0 points)
- Ex-smoker (>5 years smoke-free). (1 point)
- Current smoker or quit less than 5 years ago. (3 points)

8. Alcohol Consumption

- Rarely drink or just the occasional glass. (0 points)
- Moderate consumption (1–2 drinks a few times weekly). (1 point)
- Regular drinker (daily or heavy weekend drinking). (3 points)

Section 3: Skin Care & History

9. Current Skincare Routine

- Consistent regime with quality products including targeted actives (retinol, vitamin C, SPF, etc.). (0 points)
- Basic cleanse and moisturise. (1 point)
- Splash of water … when I remember. (3 points)

10. Childhood Sun Exposure

- Protected; minimal sunburns. (0 points)
- Occasional sunburns. (1 point)
- Multiple, severe sunburns. (3 points)

11. Skin Sensitivity

- My skin is resilient and rarely reacts. (0 points)
- Occasionally reactive to new products. (1 point)
- Highly sensitive with frequent reactions. (3 points)

12. Inflammatory Skin Conditions

- No history of inflammatory skin conditions. (0 points)
- Occasional, mild flare-ups (eczema, acne, rosacea). (1 point)
- Chronic or severe inflammatory skin issues. (3 points)

Calculate Your Score

0–8 Points: The Inflammation Optimiser

- Your inflammation risk: Low. Well done!
- Priority chapters: 1, 2, 11 & 12.
- You're already doing many things right! Focus on prevention and optimisation.

9–18 Points: The Inflammation Reducer

- Your inflammation risk: Moderate.
- Priority chapters: 3, 5, 7, 9, 11 & 12.
- You've got a good foundation but could benefit from targeted improvements.

19–26 Points: The Inflammation Transformer

- Your inflammation risk: High.
- Priority chapters: 3, 5, 6, 7, 8, 9, 11 & 12.
- Time for meaningful change with focused strategies.

27–36 Points: The Inflammation Revolutionist

- Your inflammation risk: Very High.
- Priority chapters: All – start from the beginning!
- Your skin is sending clear SOS signals. Let's address them systematically.

Your Personal Chapter Guide

High scores in questions 1–4? Start with Chapters 3, 8 & 9 to address lifestyle factors.

High scores in questions 5–8? Focus on Chapters 5, 6 & 7 to improve nutrition and internal factors.

High scores in questions 9–12? Begin with Chapters 2, 11 & 12 for skin-specific guidance.

Remember: Your skin's story isn't set in stone! Every positive change makes a difference. Retake this quiz every three months as you implement the book's strategies. Your future self (and skin!) will thank you.

AUTHOR PROFILE

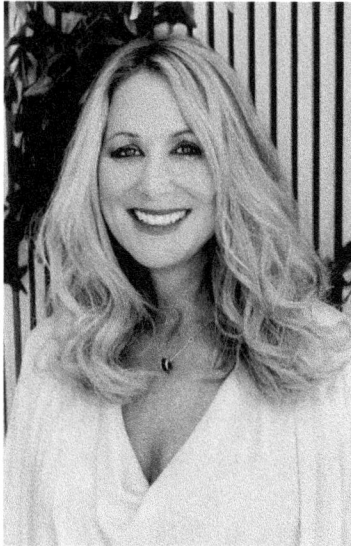

From GP and prison doctor (don't worry, she was treating the inmates not serving time!) to aesthetic industry powerhouse, Dr Victoria Manning has become one of the most respected voices in aesthetic medicine since graduating from Southampton Medical School in 1996. After discovering her passion for aesthetics in 2003, she's gone on to become a *tour de force* in the industry, collecting accolades and turning heads with her innovative techniques.

With her business partner, Dr Charlotte Woodward, she founded River Aesthetics in 2013, where their reputation for natural-looking results and cutting-edge treatments has made them the go-to clinic for those in the know. A true pioneer in collagen stimulation and thread lifting, Victoria spends much of her time treating and studying inflammatory skin conditions, bringing her medical expertise to the forefront of aesthetic treatments. Her deep understanding of skin inflammation has shaped her approach to aesthetic medicine, making her highly sought after worldwide as a trainer and speaker for leading pharmaceutical companies.

Her multiple publications in aesthetic journals have shaped industry practises, and her next venture - the innovative skincare brand, DOSED by Doctors, launching in 2026 - promises to revolutionise clinical skincare.

When she's not transforming faces, treating inflammatory conditions or training the next generation of aesthetic doctors, you'll find her in the charming New Forest town of Lymington, enjoying life's pleasures. A firm believer in practising what she preaches when it comes to ageing well, Victoria enjoys a glass of red wine - not just for its taste, but also for its beauty-boosting benefits!

Between taking her dogs for adventures, riding through the New Forest and sailing along the coast, Victoria embodies the balance of professional excellence and *joie de vivre* that has made her one of the most influential figures in aesthetic medicine today.

WHAT DID YOU THINK OF BUSTING THE CODE TO AGEING: HOW TO WIN THE INFLAMMATION GAME

A big thank you for purchasing this book. It means a lot that you chose this book specifically from such a wide range on offer. I do hope you enjoyed it.

Book reviews are incredibly important for an author. All feedback helps them improve their writing for future projects and for developing this edition. If you are able to spare a few minutes to post a review on Amazon, that would be much appreciated.

Publisher Information

rowanvale
books

Rowanvale Books provides publishing services to independent authors, writers and poets all over the globe. We deliver a personal, honest and efficient service that allows authors to see their work published, while remaining in control of the process and retaining their creativity. By making publishing services available to authors in a cost-effective and ethical way, we at Rowanvale Books hope to ensure that the local, national and international community benefits from a steady stream of good quality literature.

For more information about us, our authors or our publications, please get in touch.

www.rowanvalebooks.com
info@rowanvalebooks.com

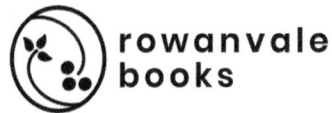

www.ingramcontent.com/pod-product-compliance
Lightning Source LLC
Chambersburg PA
CBHW042116190326
41519CB00030B/7516